A Colour Atlas of

Stroke

Cerebrovascular disease and its management

Asif Kamal
MB, BS, MRCP
Consultant Physician in Geriatric Medicine
St George's Hospital, Lincoln

Wolfe Medical Publications Ltd

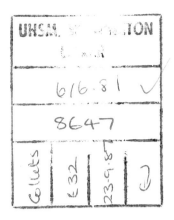
Copyright © Asif Kamal, 1987
Published by Wolfe Medical Publications Ltd, 1987
Printed by W.S. Cowell Ltd, Ipswich, England
ISBN 0 7234 0872 6

This book is one of the titles in the series of
Wolfe Medical Atlases, a series that brings
together probably the world's largest systematic
published collection of diagnostic colour
photographs.
For a full list of Atlases in the series, plus
forthcoming titles and details of our surgical,
dental and veterinary Atlases, please write to
Wolfe Medical Publications Ltd, Wolfe House,
3 Conway Street, London W1P 6HE.

General Editor, Wolfe Medical Atlases:
G. Barry Carruthers, MD(London)

CONTENTS

CONTRIBUTORS

Gillian Snowley, B.Sc (Hons), Dip. Ed., SRN, Dip. Nurs., RNT, Senior Nurse Tutor, Lincoln

Pauline Watson, Dip. COT, Senior Occupational Therapist, Sheffield

Janice Corlett, MCSP, Senior Physiotherapist, Lincoln

Lauri Softley, MCST, Senior Speech Therapist, Lincoln

Sheana Bennett, Principal Social Worker, Lincoln

Fay Killingworth, Senior Social Worker, Lincoln

ACKNOWLEDGEMENTS

I have received valuable help from numerous friends and colleagues in the preparation of this book. My thanks are due to:

The nursing staff of St George's Hospital, Lincoln, and the patients who kindly allowed me to reproduce their pictures. Dr T. Powell, Mr I. F. Lane, Mr E. G. Hale, Dr J. M. F. McClemont, Dr J. A. N. Corsellis, Dr Ariela Pomerance, Jeff Minkler, MD, Dr D. Prangnell, Dr S. Mejzner, Gillian Snowley, Lauri Softley, Jan Corlett, Pauline Watson, Derek Robinson and Peter Legat of Boehringer Ingelheim Limited, Dr Klaus Muller-Wellensiek and Jane Coffey.

I am also grateful to the following sources for permitting me to use their illustrations: Ciba-Geigy Pharmaceuticals (**1, 13, 17 to 19, 22, 26, 33, 41, 64**). Hoechst UK Ltd (**49, 142, 148**). W. Blackwood, T. C. Dodds and J. C. Sommerville, *Atlas of neuropathology*, Churchill Livingstone (**30, 62, 68, 69, 111**). Sir John Walton, *Essentials of neurology*, Pitman Publishing Ltd (**39, 210, 219**). Nottingham Medical Aids (**285, 422 to 424, 443 to 456, 457**). J. A. N. Corsellis, *Age and ageing* (**2, 25, 27**). *Echocardiography: techniques and interpretation*, Lea and Febiger, (**152, 153**). Bayer UK Ltd (**306, 307**). Farmitalia Carlo Erba Ltd, G. Weber and P. Tosi (**8a, b, c, d**). R. M. Greenhalgh and F. Clifford Rose (eds), *Progress in stroke research — 2*, Pitman Publishing Ltd (**63, 71**). Hutchison and Acheson, *Strokes — natural history, pathology and surgical treatment*, W. B. Saunders Co. Ltd (**227**). George L. Montgomery, *Textbook of pathology, Vol. 2*, Churchill Livingstone (**14, 21, 47, 65, 66, 117**). Dr Ariela Pomerance and the *British Heart Journal* (**53 to 56**). A. Schneidau and the *British Journal of Hospital Medicine* (**216 to 218**). Medical Assist Ltd (**317**). Jeff Minkler, Nervous system. In: W. A. D. Anderson (ed.), *Pathology*, 5th edn, CV Mosby Company (**23**). Boehringer Ingelheim (**9 to 12, 20, 48, 50, 52, 57, 78, 79**). John Marshall, *Management of cerebrovascular disease*, Blackwell Scientific Publications Ltd (**29, 40, 76, 80, 208**). C. D. Binnie, A. J. Rown and T. H. Gutter, *The manual of electroencephalographic technology*, Cambridge University Press (**154 to 156**). Coloplast (**314, 315**). Professor Stanley L. Robins and W. B. Saunders (**67, 81, 85, 131**). Servier Laboratories Ltd (**146**). Hoechst and Dr Klaus Muller-Wellensiek (**223 to 225**).

I would also like to acknowledge the help of various companies and organisations whose products are either mentioned in the text or appear in the pictures.

My special thanks are due to Peter Wilson and Gus de Cozar for their medical photography, and to Maureen Coffey for typing the manuscript and collecting the slides.

Asif Kamal

PREFACE

Cerebrovascular disease is a major medical problem in the advanced countries and ranks with cancer and heart disease in its prevalence. It is common in the elderly, in whom it usually presents as a stroke. In Great Britain there are about 130,000 people living, with varying disabilities, after having suffered a cerebrovascular episode. A large number of such patients are initially admitted to hospitals where, in recent years, significant advances have been made in the fields of medical management, nursing care and rehabilitation. The concept of a Stroke Unit is a comparatively new idea and will no doubt develop further in years to come.

Developments in medicine and health care have created a resurgence of interest in cerebrovascular disorders. Our knowledge about the natural history of the disease has expanded and there have been important advances in understanding risk factors, prevention, and surgical treatment. Investigative techniques, such as digital subtraction angiography, CT scanning and Doppler imaging, are progressing rapidly, providing exciting possibilities in diagnosis. Drugs are now available that will reduce platelet stickiness, and large clinical trials are in progress to determine their value in stroke prevention. Rehabilitation is not limited to splints and dreary exercises; it has developed along sound physiological principles, in which physiotherapists, occupational therapists, speech therapists and social workers play a vital part. Modern geriatric medical departments have made valuable contributions to the understanding of different types of strokes and have also pioneered the concept of multidisciplinary rehabilitation for older patients. Finally, the new progressive nursing care must be the single most important factor contributing to the better management of stroke patients.

This Atlas is an introduction to the complex subject of stroke illness. It is an attempt to link the many disciplines and specialties involved in patient management and give a broad but homogeneous picture. Throughout, the emphasis is on the treatment of stroke patients, especially the elderly, as most victims are over 65 years of age. It is intended to be used as a 'field guide' to assist in the practical management of patients who are disabled by cerebrovascular disease. It is not a comprehensive textbook (of which there are many excellent examples) and discussion of some rapidly evolving and sometimes controversial subjects, such as prevention, treatment of hypertension and physiology of cerebrovascular disease, is given only briefly. Traumatic brain disorders causing stroke-like illness are excluded. The emphasis is on the illustrations and the text is kept to the minimum.

I hope that this Atlas will be of value to all those who are concerned with treatment and rehabilitation of stroke patients, especially non-specialist medical and paramedical staff.

Asif Kamal

INTRODUCTION: DEFINITION AND INCIDENCE

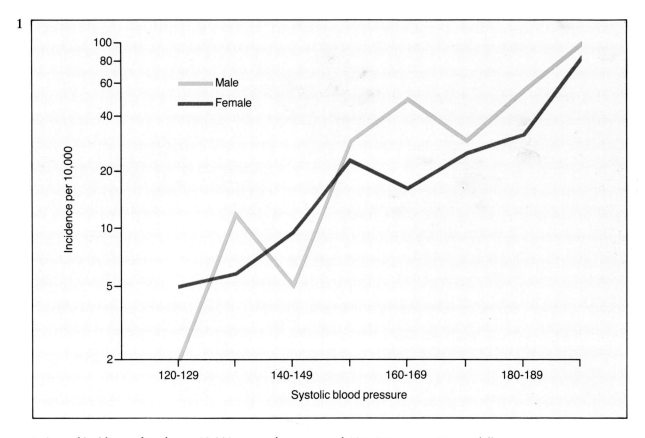

1 Annual incidence of stroke per 10,000 men and women aged 45 to 74 years on 18-year follow-up.

A stroke is characterised by a focal neurological deficit caused by a local disturbance in the blood supply to the brain: its onset is usually abrupt but may extend over a few hours or longer.

Cerebrovascular disease is one of the most frequent causes of morbidity and mortality, especially with advancing years. Strokes can occur at any age but the incidence rises rapidly in the elderly. In Britain 16% of the population are over 65 years of age and the proportion is continuing to increase. It is therefore not surprising that most stroke patients tend to be elderly. The annual incidence rate in Britain is just under 2 per 1,000 population. For people aged 75 years and over, the annual incidence rate per 1,000 population is about 47.4. In North America, stroke is the third most common cause of death, with an incidence rate per 1,000 of 1.48 in males and 1.34 in females. In those aged 75 to 84 years this increases to 17.13. In Great Britain there are about 130,000 people surviving after a stroke and in the USA there are 2 million.

There is no significant difference in the incidence of strokes between males and females, but as females tend to live longer than males in most western countries, a higher proportion of stroke patients aged over 65 years are female. The chances of developing a cerebral infarct by the age of 70 years is about 1 in 20.

In Britain, an average general practitioner will see about five new patients with stroke each year, and will have 15 to 20 patients on his list who have had a stroke some time in the past and are living in the community. Around 75% of patients with acute strokes are admitted to hospital and of these about 40% are discharged. A typical District General Hospital will have about 500 stroke cases in its catchment area each year, of whom 250 will be severely disabled. About 50% of patients die within 3 to 5 years of an acute stroke, most dying within 1 month of the acute episode. Within 15 years, over 65% of patients will have had another stroke. The mortality in the early stages is influenced by several factors, including the pathology of the lesion: it may range from 92% for cerebral haemorrhage to 36% for cerebral thrombosis.

The long-term outlook for survivors depends upon the availability of modern rehabilitation and the quality of home care. It is difficult to predict the early prognosis in stroke survivors. Up to 30% of patients may be permanently disabled. In the Framingham survey[1] about half the survivors had motor problems, one-third had speech disorders and one-quarter had sensory deficits. However, with intensive rehabilitation and a good follow-up programme, it may be possible for up to 36% of patients to achieve a useful level of independence and activity.

The exact incidence of the pathology of lesions causing strokes is difficult to determine and results of various clinical and post-mortem studies have been conflicting. Thromboembolism is commoner than haemorrhage, but atheroma in cerebral arteries may be widespread and causes difficulty in interpreting the exact pathology. Under the age of 35 years, subarachnoid haemorrhage causes nearly 50% of all strokes, but over the age of 70 years this becomes infrequent.

The significance of racial origin in the incidence of stroke is unclear. However, there is increased incidence in American negroes and the Japanese.

RISK FACTORS

The risk factors for cerebrovascular disease are the same as those for hypertension and atheroma. Both risk factors and incidence of stroke increase with age.

Blood pressure

The World Health Organisation defines hypertension as a systolic blood pressure of 160 mm Hg or above, and a diastolic blood pressure of 95 mm Hg or above, on repeated measurements. Raised blood pressure is the most important risk factor for cerebrovascular disease. In elderly patients, isolated systolic hypertension is also significant. It is estimated that in hypertensives there is a fourfold increase in the incidence of stroke, particularly as a result of cerebral infarction and cerebral haemorrhage. Good control of moderate and severe hypertension reduces the incidence of stroke. The Medical Research Council's mild hypertension trial has shown that by treating middle-aged people the stroke rate was reduced.[2] There were 60 strokes in the treated group and 109 in the placebo group, giving rates of 1.4 and 2.6 per 1,000 patient years of observation respectively. The work of the European Working Party on High Blood Pressure in the Elderly has shown that treatment has no effect on overall mortality or cerebral vascular mortality, but non-fatal cerebrovascular events were significantly reduced by about 50%.[3]

Heart disease

About 5% of strokes are caused by emboli arising from the heart. Cerebral embolism occurs with mitral stenosis, subacute bacterial endocarditis, mural thrombosis after myocardial infarction, cardiomyopathy, prolapsed mitral valve, atrial myxoma and prosthetic heart valves.

Transient cardiac arrhythmias can be detected by 24-hour ambulatory cardiac monitoring. These can sometimes cause minor strokes and other cerebral symptoms, especially in elderly patients.

Transient ischaemic attacks (TIAs)

TIAs are considered to be harbingers of a major stroke. Up to 40% of all patients who have a TIA go on to develop a stroke within 2 years. Carotid artery TIAs are more liable to result in a stroke than those in the vertebrobasilar territory.

Genetic factors

Family history is important, as some families are more prone to hypertension than others. Racial differences are notable, for example American negroes are more susceptible to vascular disease than whites. Japanese have a high incidence of cerebral haemorrhage.

Smoking

Smoking promotes atheroma. It also causes vasoconstriction and increases blood viscosity. The platelets become more sticky and fibrinolytic activity is decreased. These various factors increase both atherogenesis and the tendency to thrombosis.

Diabetes mellitus

Diabetes and hypertension tend to coexist, and diabetes is commoner in stroke patients than in the normal population of similar age and sex.

Contraceptive pill

The oral contraceptive pill increases the risk of stroke amongst young women of child-bearing age. There is also increased incidence of venous thromboembolism.

Age and sex

The incidence of stroke rises with age. The chance of developing a stroke by the age of 75 years is about 1 in 20. Cerebrovascular disease tends to affect men at younger ages and women after the menopause. It is thought that female hormones have a protective effect against arteriosclerosis.

Obesity

The relationship between stroke and obesity is unclear. Raised blood lipids in obese subjects may cause atheroma in later life, thus contributing to the development of a stroke.

Socioeconomic status

The incidence of stroke is high in the lower socioeconomic groups. However, this observation is relevant only to western 'civilized' countries.

Other risk factors

Other risk factors for stroke include sickle cell disease, increased blood viscosity, e.g. polycythaemia, syphilis, extremes of climate and temperature, and hyperlipidaemia.

Strokes in children are rare but may occur with congenital abnormalities of cerebral blood vessels, brain damage during difficult labour, infection, malnutrition, sickle cell disease, meningitis or trauma, or may be idiopathic.

PATHOLOGY

Atheroma is the main pathological feature in cerebrovascular disease. Its prevalence increases with advancing age, when there is arterial intimal thickening and elastic degeneration. The vessels dilate, elongate and become tortuous. Even in the absence of overt atheroma the intima and media show increased deposition of lipids, lipoproteins and calcium salts.

The aetiology of arteriosclerosis is multifactorial and the subject of much research and controversy. However, there is an association with the following:

- Stress.
- Hypertension.
- Diabetes mellitus.
- Advancing age.
- Diet rich in lipids and cholesterol and low in fibre.
- Smoking.

Arteriosclerosis affects the large and medium-sized arteries. Arterioles with a diameter less than 0.3 mm are not involved. All major arteries may be affected but the condition shows a predilection for the vessels to the heart and brain. The arteriosclerotic plaques tend to occur at points of mechanical stress, such as bifurcations. Fatty streaks in the intima are the earliest manifestation, and in elderly subjects these can be found in most large arteries. These then progress through the stages of lipid accumulation, overgrowth of fibrous tissue, plaque formation, calcification and eventually confluent atheroma. Atherosclerotic plaques are capable of initiating thrombosis within the vessels, which will result in vessel occlusion. Increased platelet adhesiveness is crucial in initiating thrombosis — two substances, thromboxane and prostacyclin, are important in this respect. Ulceration of an atherosclerotic plaque initiates a sequence of events resulting in thrombosis.

Effects of atherosclerosis

- Narrowing of arterial lumen.
- Complete occlusion, thrombosis.
- Arterial dilatation.
- Aneurysm formation.
- Ulceration of plaque.
- Rupture causing haemorrhage.

These effects of atheroma will give rise to ischaemic heart disease, cerebral infarction and haemorrhage, and peripheral vascular disease.

Collateral circulation (see illustrations of cerebral circulation)

Congenital anomalies of the circle of Willis are common, resulting in abnormalities of collateral cerebral circulation. The circle of Willis with normal configuration is present in 15 to 40% of people. Abnormalities may be seen in up to 46%. The size of a cerebral infarct produced by thromboembolic occlusion of an artery will depend on the state of collateral circulation.

Cerebral blood flow (CBF)

Cerebral neurones can function only with a constant supply of oxygen and glucose. This requires an adequate cerebral blood flow. The most important regulator of CBF is the $PaCO_2$: a rise in $PaCO_2$ increases the flow, and a fall reduces the flow. A rise in blood pressure stimulates cerebrovascular resistance and a drop in blood pressure causes a drop in resistance, so that CBF remains constant. This ability of CBF to remain constant is called autoregulation. It operates by constricting or dilating cerebral arterioles. Autoregulation is impaired in hypertensive patients so that a small fall in blood pressure may lead to a dangerous fall in CBF. This must be borne in mind when treating these patients with antihypertensive drugs. Autoregulation may also be affected by chronic respiratory disease, atheroma of arteries in the neck and by ageing itself. Elderly patients with defective autoregulation are susceptible to faints and falls.

2 Circle of Willis from an elderly subject showing no evidence of atheroma.

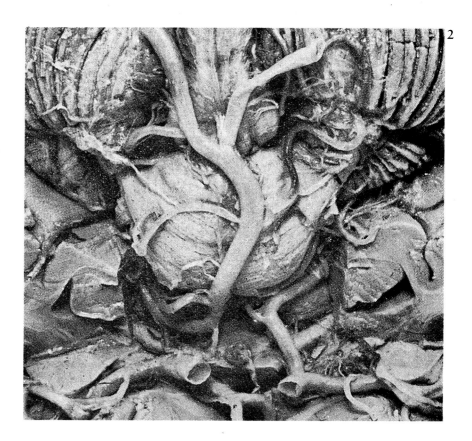
2

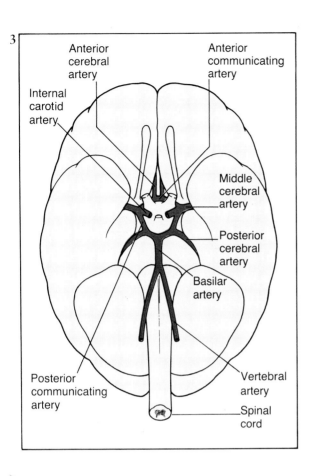

3

3 Circle of Willis showing normal configuration. This is present in only 15 to 40% of people. Abnormalities may be seen in up to 46%, with consequent abnormalities of collateral cerebral circulation.

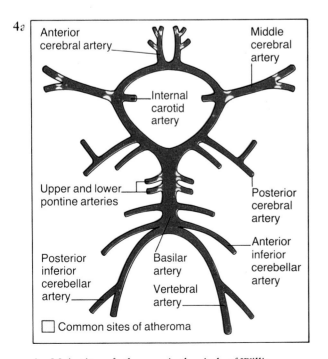

4a Main sites of atheroma in the circle of Willis.

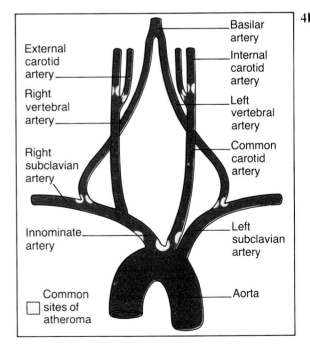

4b Sites of atheroma in the aortic arch and great vessels.

5 Major arterial territories of the brain — side view.

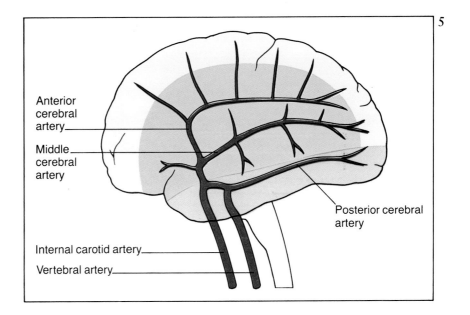

Anterior cerebral artery

Middle cerebral artery

Posterior cerebral artery

Internal carotid artery

Vertebral artery

6 Cross-section of cerebral hemisphere to show territories of main cerebral arteries.

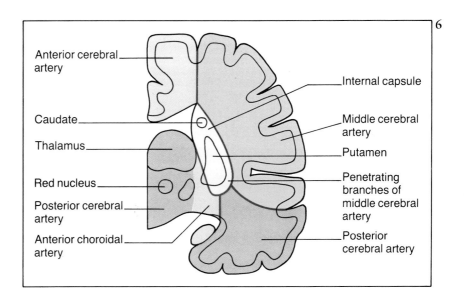

Anterior cerebral artery

Internal capsule

Caudate

Middle cerebral artery

Thalamus

Putamen

Red nucleus

Penetrating branches of middle cerebral artery

Posterior cerebral artery

Anterior choroidal artery

Posterior cerebral artery

7 Cross-section of arterial wall showing changes of early atheroma.

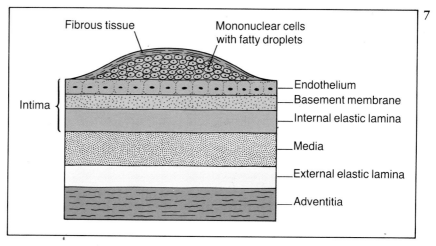

Fibrous tissue

Mononuclear cells with fatty droplets

Endothelium

Basement membrane

Intima

Internal elastic lamina

Media

External elastic lamina

Adventitia

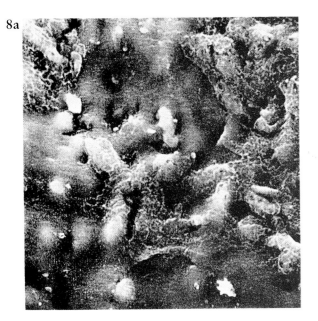

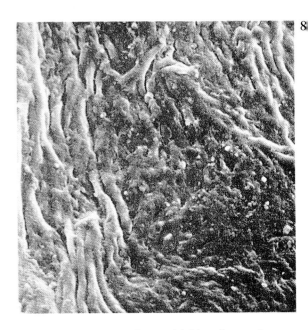

8 Scanning electron microscope pictures of guineapig aorta in experimental cholesterol atherogenesis after 12 months on a high-cholesterol diet. **8a** The intimal surface is covered by an amorphous lining, almost effacing the intimal fold design. Note the trapped blood corpuscles.

8b The normal relief of intimal folds is flattened.

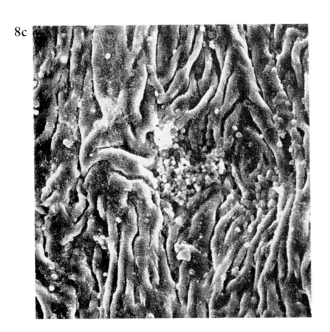

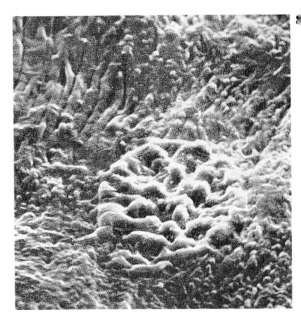

8c Accumulation of blood corpuscles against a cluster of markedly protruding intimal folds.

8d Definite evidence of an atheromatous plaque in an area with flattened and depressed intimal folds.

9 Platelets, fibrin and red blood corpuscles in the early stages of thrombosis.

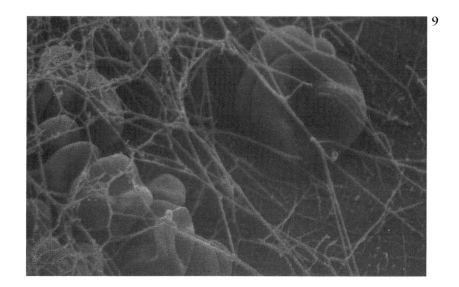

10 Close-up of wall of a large artery. In the lower part of the picture an arteriosclerotic plaque and some thrombi can be seen.

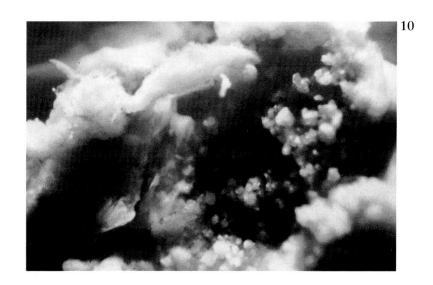

11 Large artery with severe atheromatous changes and numerous thrombi.

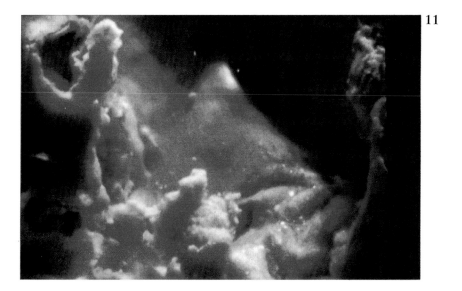

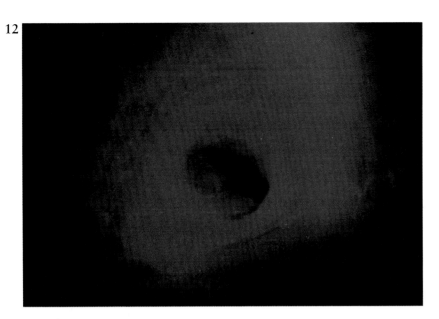

12 Severe atheromatous changes in the aorta. Thrombotic masses are partially occluding the vessel.

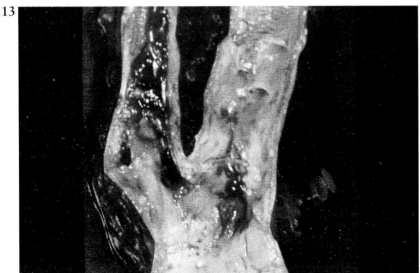

13 Intimal atheroma in a patient with prolonged hypertension.

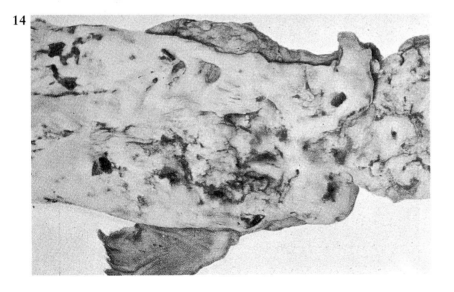

14 Advanced aortic atheroma. The intimal surface is rough because of atheromatous plaques and ulcers.

15 Plain x-ray of the chest showing unfolded aorta caused by long-standing hypertension and arteriosclerosis — a frequent finding in elderly patients.

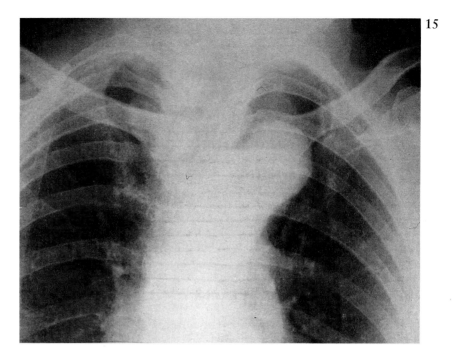

16 Calcified aortic knuckle — a frequent finding in elderly stroke patients with long-standing hypertension.

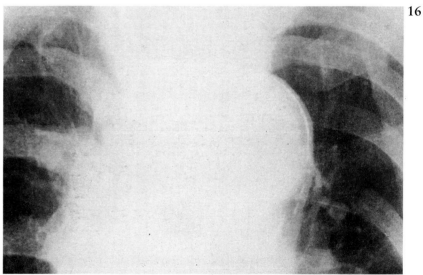

17 Hypertrophy of the muscular arteriolar wall in a patient with prolonged hypertension.

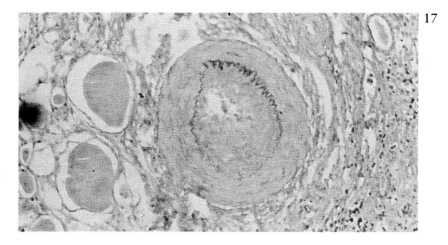

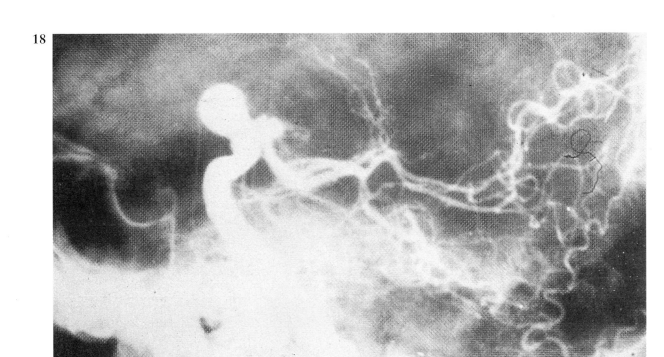

18 Increased arteriolar tortuosity in a patient with prolonged hypertension.

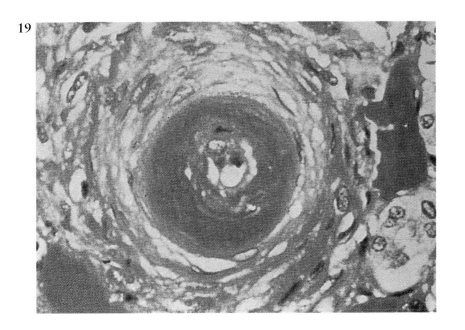

19 Narrowing of the lumen in a patient with chronic hypertension.

Causes of strokes

Most strokes are caused by cerebral infarction or cerebral haemorrhage. Atherothromboembolic brain infarction accounts for about 80% of all strokes.

I Cerebral infarction.

   a) Cerebral thrombosis.

   b) Cerebral embolism.

II Cerebral haemorrhage.

   a) Primary cerebral haemorrhage.

   b) Subarachnoid haemorrhage.

Causes of cerebral thrombosis

1 Atheroma — especially in hypertension, diabetes and smoking.
2 Arteritis (inflammatory disease of the arteries) — meningovascular syphilis, polyarteritis, temporal arteritis, typhus, Takayasu's disease, Moya-Moya disease.
3 Cerebral thrombophlebitis — secondary to infection of ear, paranasal sinus, face, etc.
4 Haematological disorders — polycythaemia, sickle cell disease, myeloma, thrombocythaemia, thrombotic thrombocytopenic purpura, paroxysmal nocturnal haemoglobinuria, dehydration.
5 Trauma to carotid arteries and arteriography.
6 Dissecting aortic aneurysm.
7 Severe systemic hypotension — e.g. hypotensive cerebral infarction in the elderly.
8 Middle cerebral artery thrombosis in closed head injury.
9 Hypothermia in the elderly.

Causes of cerebral embolism

a) Cardiac origin
 1 Myocardial infarction with mural thrombus (4 to 15%).
 2 Bacterial endocarditis.
 3 Atrial fibrillation with mitral stenosis.
 4 Cardiac valve disease or prosthesis (mitral valve prolapse).
 5 Non-bacterial thrombotic endocarditis.
 6 Paradoxical embolism with congenital heart disease.
 7 Cardiomyopathy.
 8 Left atrial myxoma.
 9 Trichinosis.
10 Complication of cardiac surgery.
11 Sick sinus syndrome — less than 2% of elderly stroke patients have this syndrome.
12 Mitral annulus calcification in the elderly.

b) Non-cardiac origin
 1 Atheroma of aorta and carotid arteries.
 2 Thrombus in pulmonary vein.
 3 Fat, air or tumour embolism.
 4 Complications of neck surgery.

Causes of intracranial haemorrhage

1 Vascular anomaly.
  Aneurysm.
  Angioma.
2 Hypertension.
3 Haemorrhagic disorders, anticoagulants.
4 Tumours.
5 Trauma.
6 Septic embolism, mycotic aneurysm.
7 Haemorrhagic infarction.
8 Inflammatory disease of the arteries and veins.

Cerebral thrombosis

The common sites of atheroma and thrombosis are the internal carotid artery, bifurcation of the middle cerebral artery, at the junction of vertebral and basilar arteries, posterior cerebral artery, anterior cerebral artery and vertebral arteries at their origins from the subclavian. Occlusion of the penetrating branches will produce tiny infarcts that eventually become cystic and are called 'lacunae'. In most cases cerebral infarction occurs as a result of occlusion of a single feeding cerebral artery.

Cerebral embolism

Most emboli arise from the heart or the large arteries and lodge in a cerebral vessel. The origins of the carotid arteries from the aorta are a major site of atheromatous plaques, and either thrombus or atherosclerotic debris can become detached from the plaque and be carried up into the cerebral circulation. In many cases it is impossible to differentiate between thrombosis and embolism.

Transient cerebral ischaemic attacks (TIAs) are a form of cerebral micro-embolism and are discussed later (see chapter on clinical manifestations).

Cerebral infarction

Cerebral infarction results from severe ischaemia caused by thrombosis or embolism. The size of the infarct will depend upon the territory supplied by the blocked blood vessel and the adequacy of collateral circulation. Sometimes infarction occurs as a result of a sudden fall in blood pressure, which reduces the cerebral blood flow and gives rise to infarction in the so-called 'boundary zones' (watershed infarction) in the cerebral circulation. This happens particularly in elderly patients who may have both severe postural hypotension and defective autoregulation. Postural hypotension in the elderly can occur as a result of abnormal baroreceptor reflexes, diminished cardiac output, drugs, parkinsonism and hyponatraemia. With occlusion of the blood vessel, the area of brain beyond becomes pale, soft and swollen. The neurones die and the demarcation between grey and white matter becomes blurred. Infarcts may become haemorrhagic if blood leaks into the area. Eventually the infarct shrinks. The cerebral oedema following infarction results from astrocytic swelling and accumulation of extracellar fluid. After about 6 weeks, the infarct begins to cavitate and the end result is a cystic cavity. The surface of the brain overlying the infarct is depressed and the adjacent ventricle may be distorted and dilated.

Brains of elderly patients who have had several strokes may show evidence of many small infarcts with some cerebral atrophy and dilatation of the ventricles — such patients may have had features of multi-infarct dementia.

Cerebral haemorrhage

a) **Primary intracerebral haemorrhage**
Hypertension
Vascular malformations
Micro-aneurysms of Charcot and Bouchard
Rupture of mycotic aneurysm
Cerebral tumours
Haemorrhagic disorders

b) **Subarachnoid haemorrhage**
Congenital berry aneurysms
Congenital vascular malformations
Haemorrhagic disorders

Primary intracerebral haemorrhage usually occurs with hypertension, which causes direct damage to the arterial wall. Sometimes there are multiple micro-infarcts and haemorrhages in the subcortical areas, which give rise to the clinical syndrome of multi-infarct dementia. Small bleeds may occur from micro-aneurysms (Charcot and Bouchard) under 2 mm in diameter, situated on the perforating arteries. Large cerebral haemorrhage causes destruction of the brain tissue. There is also oedema and frequently brain stem compression. These features are responsible for the deteriorating level of consciousness and the poor prognosis.

Subarachnoid haemorrhage occurs usually from a berry aneurysm or an arteriovenous anomaly. Berry aneurysms are 2 to 3 mm in diameter and are found around the circle of Willis; 90% of these aneurysms are caused by congenital weakness of the arterial wall in the subarachnoid space. When rupture occurs the blood pours out into the subarachnoid space and some of it leaks into the brain substance.

20 Large well-organised thrombus extending into the vessel.

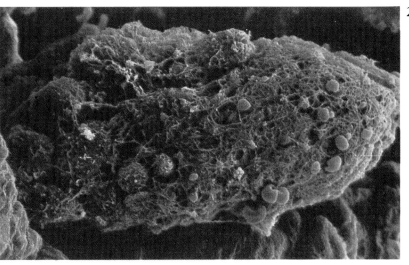

21 Atheroma of cerebral artery narrowing the lumen.

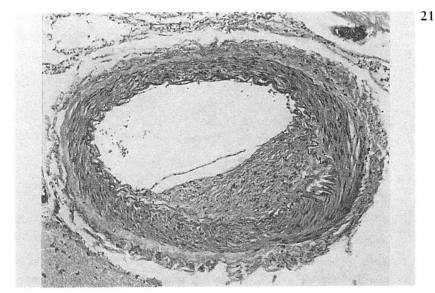

22 Section of an occluded intracranial vessel.

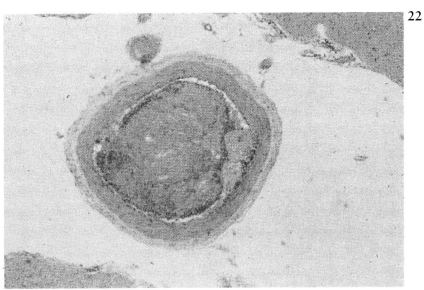

23 Thrombosis of basilar artery with infarction of the pons.

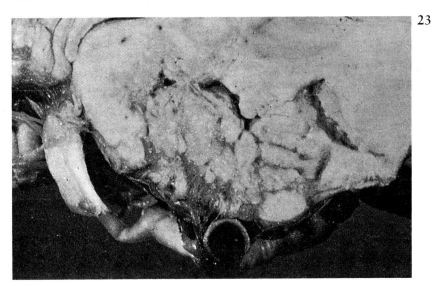

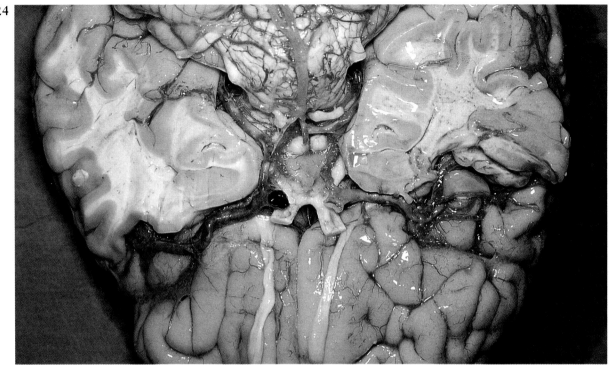

24 Left internal carotid artery thrombosis.

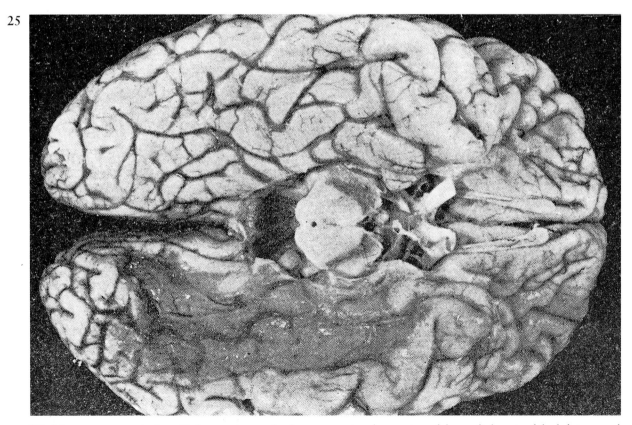

25 **Atheromatous occlusion of left posterior cerebral artery** causing destruction of the medial parts of the left temporal lobe and the under-surface of the occipital lobe.

26 Right internal carotid artery thrombosis with accompanying oedema and swelling of the right hemisphere.

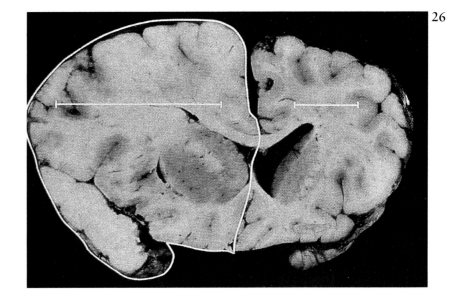

27 Severe cerebral atheroma. The arrows point to areas of infarction and softening. The left middle cerebral artery is grossly thickened.

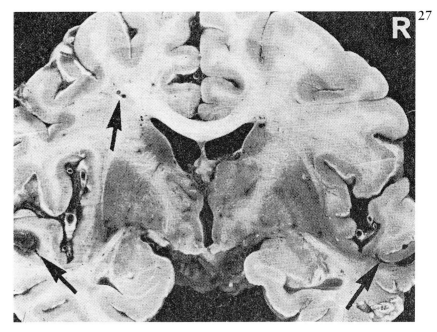

28 Cerebral infarction. Isotope scan showing large wedge-shaped area of increased uptake in the right hemisphere.

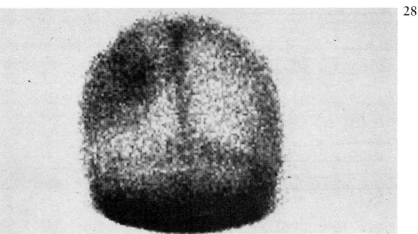

29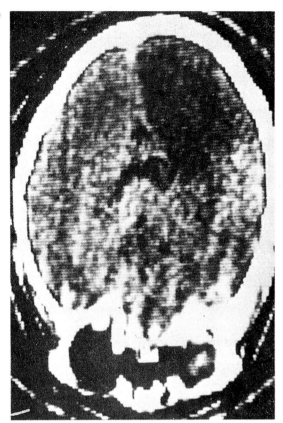

29 CT scan showing infarction in the left occipital lobe.

30

30 Anterior view of a coronal slice of brain in a case of hemiplegia. Many years back, the patient had suffered athero-sclerotic occlusion of the right middle cerebral artery.

31 Liquefactive infarct of the basal ganglia.

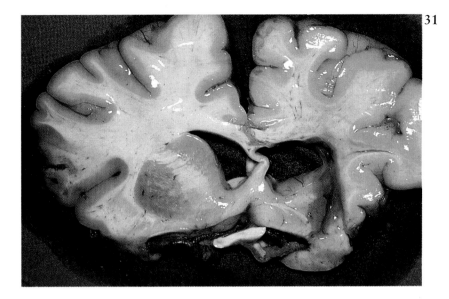

32 Slice of brain tissue showing recent infarct.

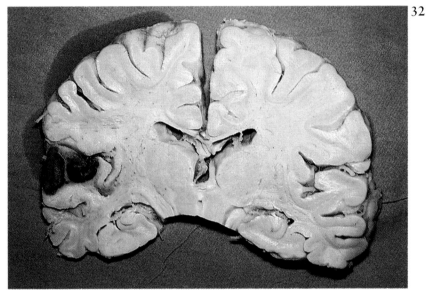

33 Occlusion of intracerebral arterioles giving rise to lacunae.

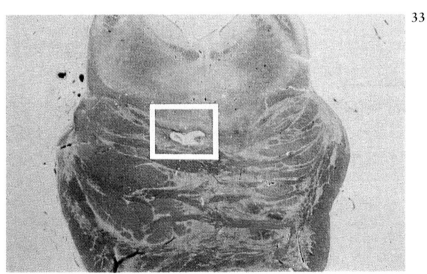

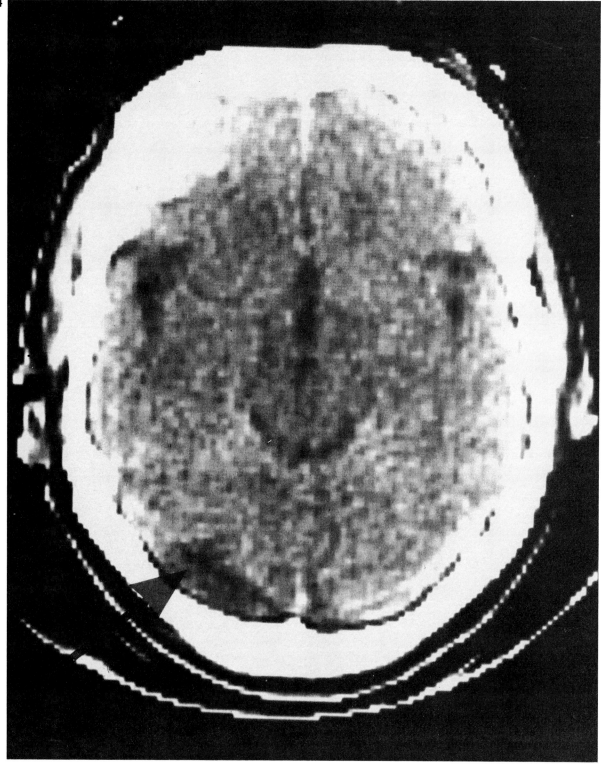

34 CT scan showing area of reduced attenuation lying superior over the posterior aspect of the left cerebellar hemisphere. This is caused by surface collection of CSF, possibly as a result of atrophy of the left cerebellar hemisphere. This may represent the end result of a cerebellar infarct.

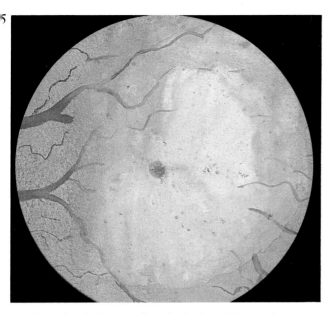

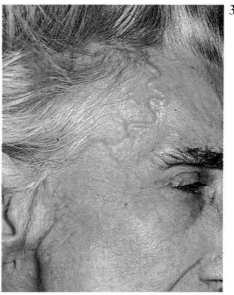

35 **Central retinal artery thrombosis.** Artist's impression of the ophthalmoscopic view of the fundus, showing pallor of the retina except at the fovea centralis, where the pinkness of the choroidal circulation is still seen as a 'cherry-red spot'.

36 **Temporal arteritis.** The patient had unilateral headache, tenderness over the right temporal region and a high ESR. There is a danger of sudden blindness from retinal artery thrombosis.

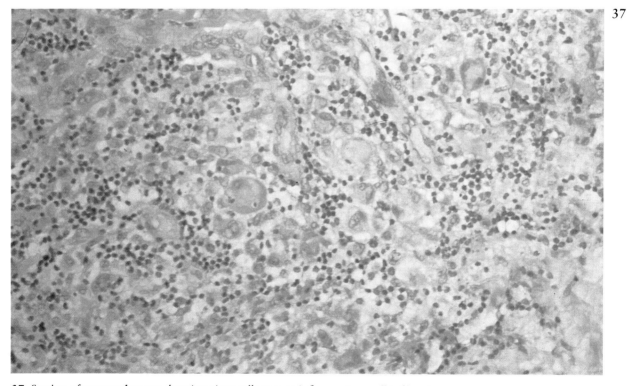

37 **Section of temporal artery** showing giant cells among inflammatory cell infiltration.

38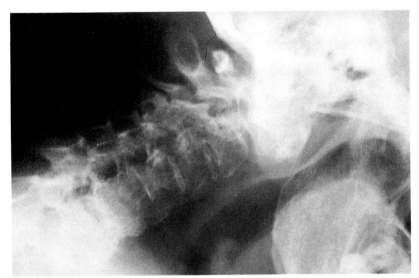

38 Degenerative changes in the cervical spine can contribute to vertebrobasilar ischaemia. This x-ray shows cervical spondylosis.

39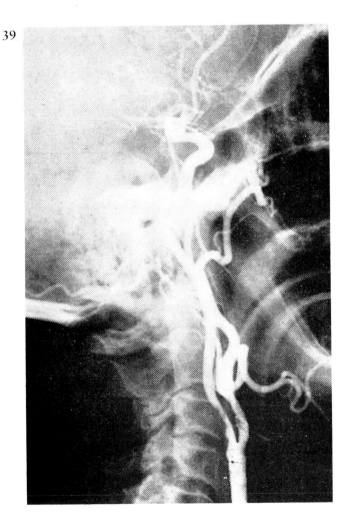

39 Carotid arteriogram showing stenosis at the origin of the internal carotid artery.

40 Atheromatous stenosis of the vertebral artery with friable platelet thrombus. Such a patient may present with transient ischaemic attacks in the vertebrobasilar territory.

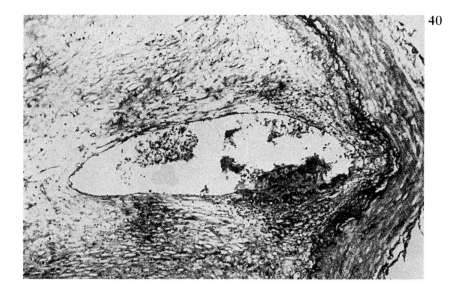

41 Rouleau formation of red blood cells caused by decreased blood flow rate and increased viscosity. Cerebral thrombosis can occur in such patients, who may have underlying myeloma, polycythaemia, dehydration or hypothermia.

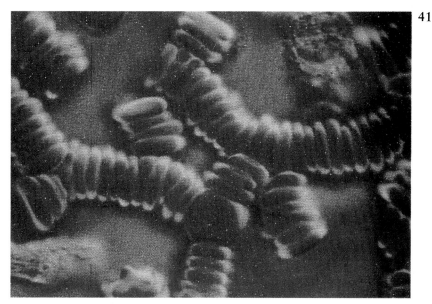

42 Sickle cell anaemia crises may give rise to cerebral thrombosis. This illustration shows typical sickling of the red blood cells.

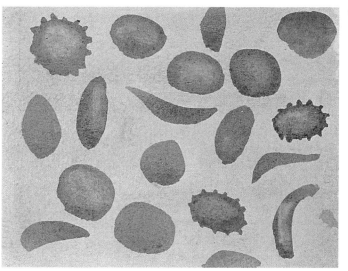

43

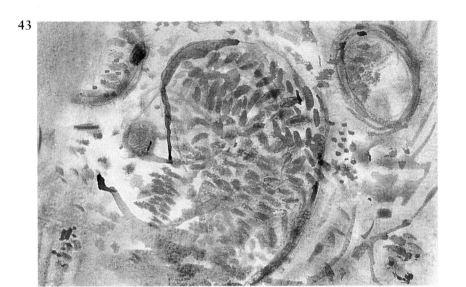

43 Cerebral capillary occluded by sickle cell thrombus. Artist's impression.

44

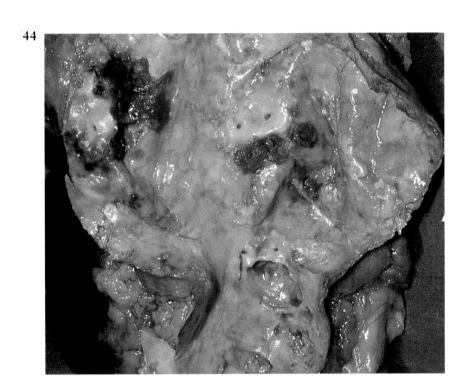

44 Aortic aneurysm with atheromatous changes.

45 Fragment of bone marrow
in a smear from a case of
polycythaemia rubra vera.
There is extreme
hypercellularity, absence of fat
spaces and great excess of
megakaryocytes. Polycythaemia
is a well-recognised cause of
cerebral thrombosis.

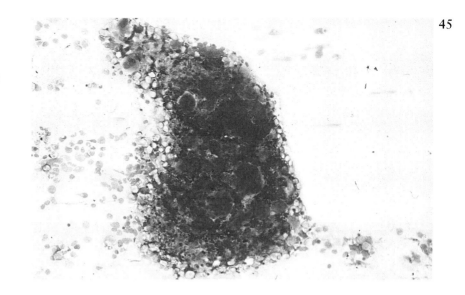

**46 Poor dental hygiene in a
case of bacterial endocarditis.**
The patient developed cerebral
embolism.

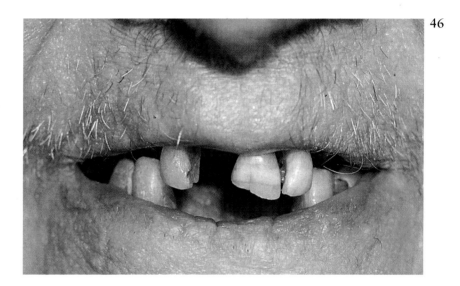

47 Bacterial endocarditis
showing friable valvular
vegetations, which are likely to
give rise to cerebral embolism.

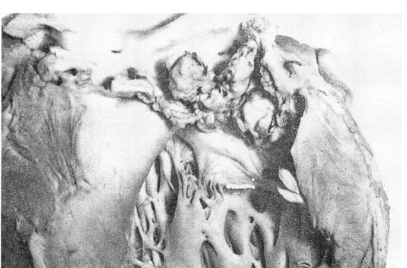

48

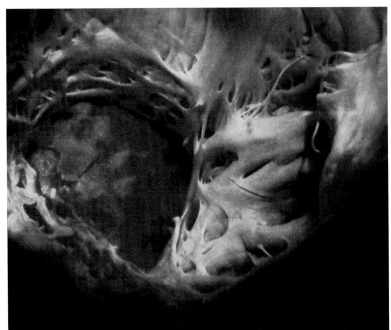

48 Thrombus in the apical part of the heart close to freshly infarcted areas of myocardium.

49

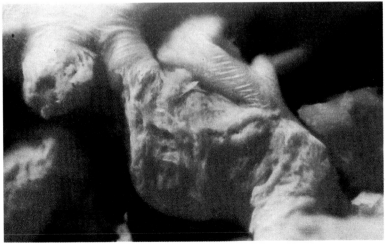

I   II   III   VR   VL   VF

V₁   V₂   V₃   V₄   V₅   V₆

49 ECG trace of anterior myocardial infarction. Cerebral embolism may occur from a mural thrombus. There are Q waves in VL and in V_1 to V_4, ST elevation in VL and in V_2 to V_5, and early T wave inversion in V_3 to V_4.

50

50 Close-up of a small thrombus wedged between the trabeculae of the heart.

51 X-ray of the chest in mitral stenosis. Note the prominence of the left atrium. Combination of atrial fibrillation and mitral stenosis can cause cerebral embolism.

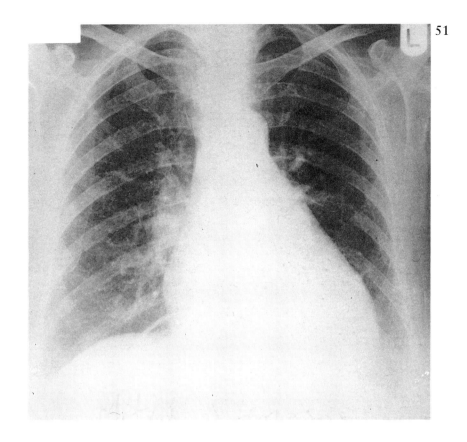

52 Thrombus in the left atrium of a patient with mitral stenosis.

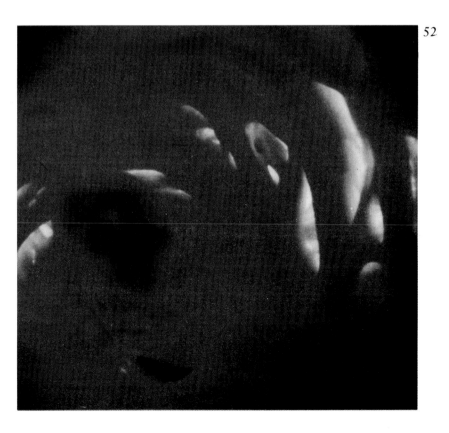

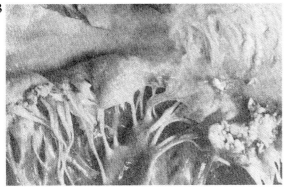

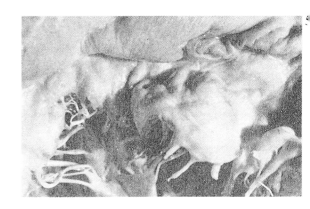

53 **Floppy mitral valve.** Opened left side of the heart showing ballooning, more marked in the posterior cusp, with large vegetations. This patient had congestive cardiac failure, a loud apical pansystolic murmur and renal and cerebral embolism.

54 **Floppy mitral valve** showing three ruptured chordae tendinae attached to the ballooned and thickened posterior cusp.

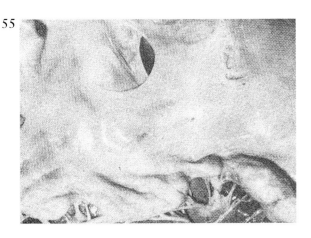

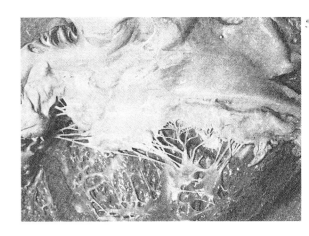

55 **Part of opened left side of the heart showing an atrial septal defect and ballooning deformity of both mitral cusps.** This is from a woman aged 75 years who was admitted with recurrent hemiplegia.

56 **Opened left side of heart showing ballooned and floppy mitral valve.** Spurs of calcium extend from the ring and distort the posterior cusp. Small patches of endocardial fibrosis are seen high on the posterior wall of the ventricle.

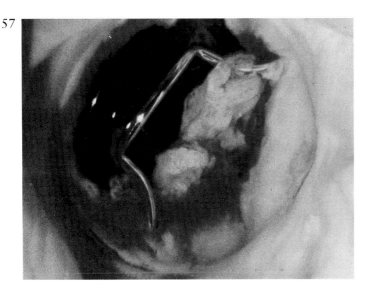

57 **Thrombus lodged on an artificial heart valve.**

58 X-ray of the chest showing enlarged heart in cardiomyopathy. The patient presented with a sudden hemiplegia.

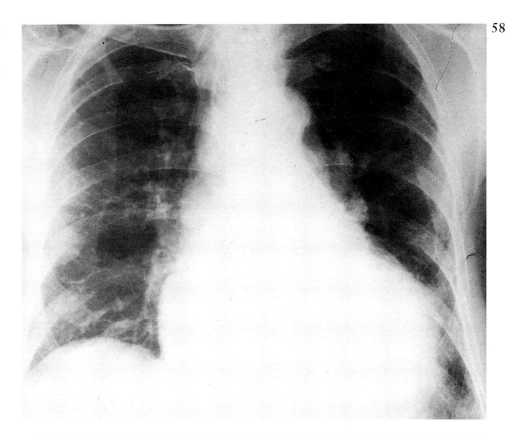

59 Aortic aneurysm involving the descending aorta and caused by arteriosclerosis. Note streaks of calcification in the vessel wall.

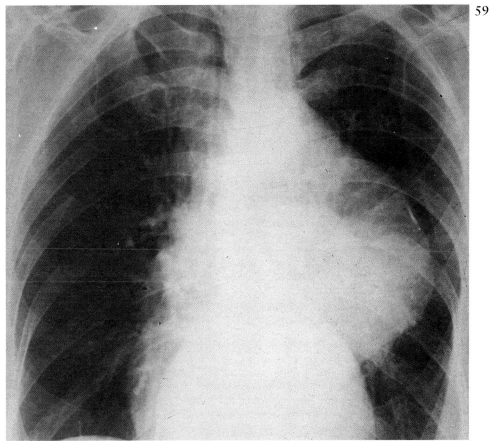

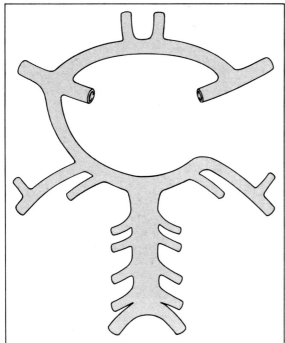

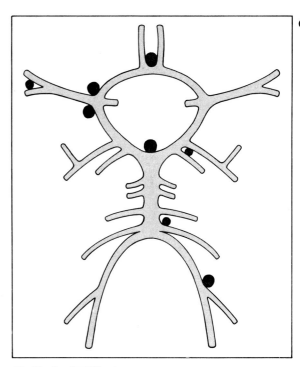

60 **Circle of Willis showing congenital absence of the right posterior communicating artery.** The effects of cerebral thrombosis are considerably more serious in such patients, because of defective collateral circulation in the brain.

61 Circle of Willis showing main sites of saccular aneurysms.

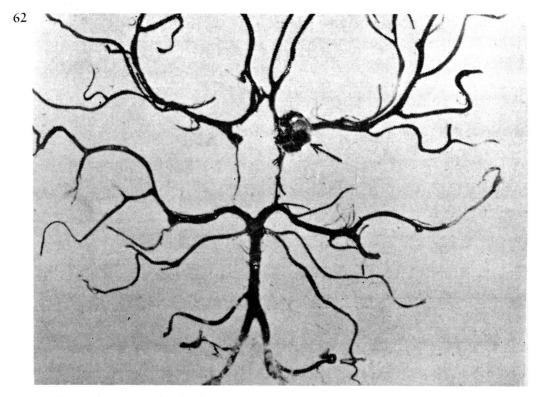

62 **Dissected out circle of Willis** showing a saccular aneurysm at the origin of the ophthalmic artery from the internal carotid artery.

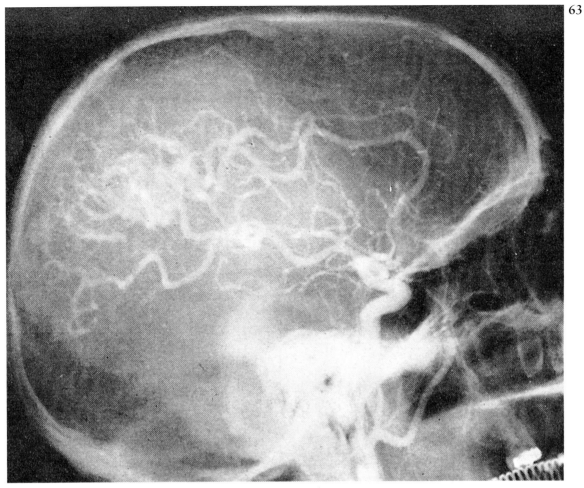

63 Carotid arteriogram showing an arteriovenous malformation in the posterior occipital region.

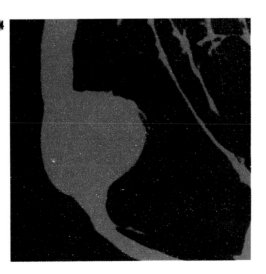

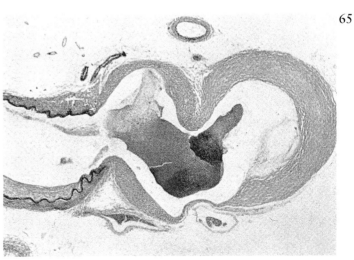

64 **Micro-aneurysm of Charcot-Bouchard type,** often responsible for primary cerebral haemorrhage.

65 **Congenital 'berry' aneurysm.** These can cause subarachnoid haemorrhage. The size varies from 2 mm to 3 cm.

66

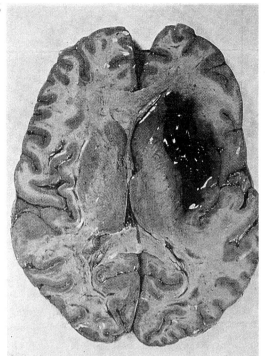

66 Massive intracerebral haemorrhage.

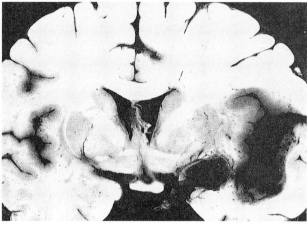

67 Meningocerebral haemorrhage.

68

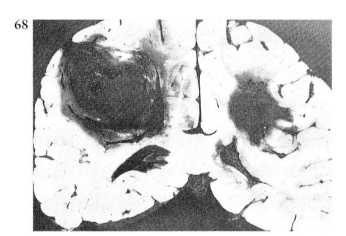

68 Multiple cerebral haemorrhages.

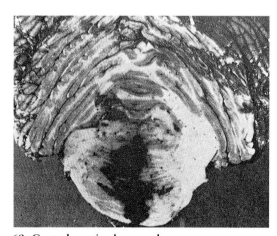

69 Central pontine haemorrhage.

70 CT scan showing large mass in the left frontal lobe with high attenuation and surrounding zone of reduced attenuation. Moderate compression of the frontal horn of the left lateral ventricle is seen. The appearances are those of a haematoma probably 7 to 10 days old.

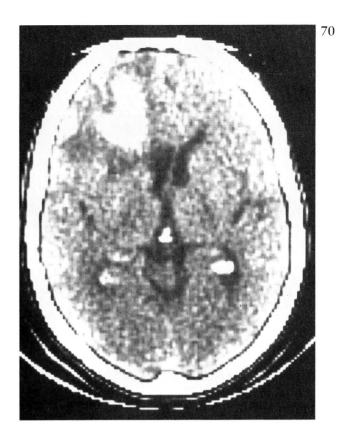

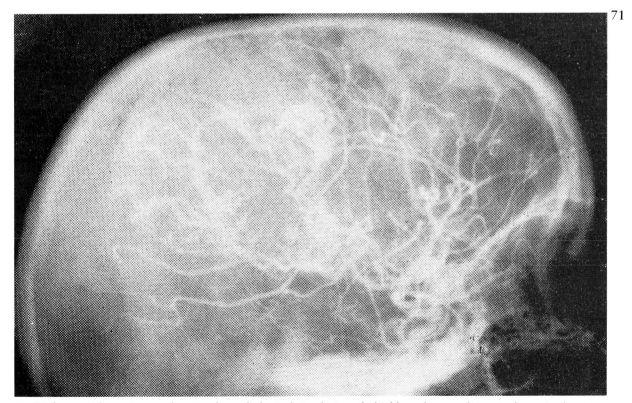

71 Right carotid arteriogram showing the pathological circulation of a highly malignant glioma in the parietal region. Haemorrhage within the tumour can present as stroke.

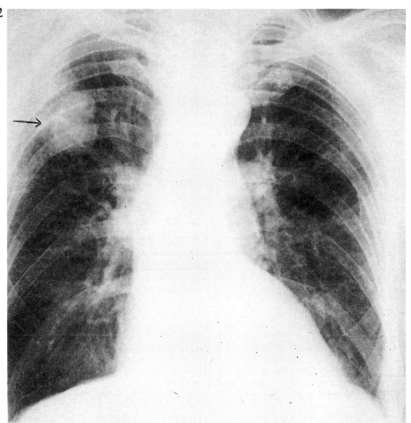

72 Plain x-ray of the chest showing a tumour in the right upper lobe. Cerebral metastases from such a tumour can give rise to a stroke-like picture.

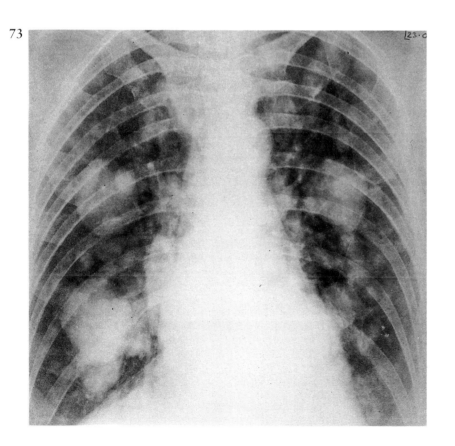

73 Plain x-ray of the chest showing multiple pulmonary metastases from an excised melanoma on the hand. The patient had cerebral metastases too and presented with hemiparesis and dysphasia.

74 Section of brain showing a large astrocytoma in the left hemisphere. The patient will have right-sided hemiplegia.

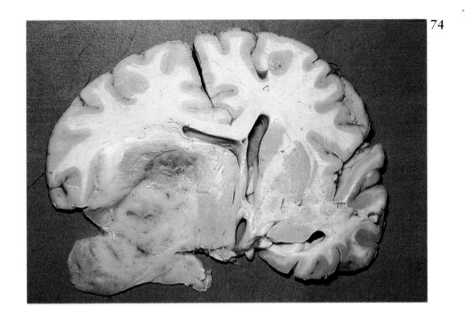

75 Multiple myeloma is one of the haematological disorders that can cause stroke. The illustration shows the typical large myeloma cells with eccentrically placed nuclei.

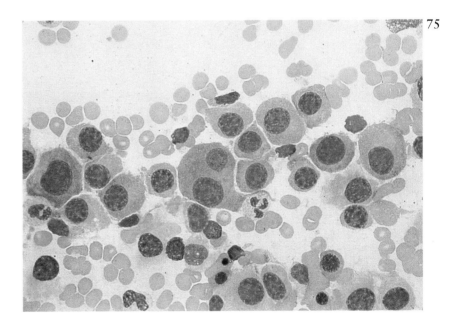

CLINICAL MANIFESTATIONS

Cerebrovascular disease may present with a number of different clinical pictures, the most frequent being the syndrome of sudden-onset stroke with hemiplegia.

Clinical types

- Major strokes — infarction and haemorrhage.
- Subarachnoid haemorrhage.
- Minor strokes.
- Stroke-in-evolution.
- Transient ischaemic attacks (TIAs).
- Multi-infarct dementia.
- Boundary zone infarction.
- Intracranial thrombophlebitis and cerebral venous thrombosis.
- Unruptured aneurysms.
- Arteriovenous malformation.
- Cerebellar haemorrhage.
- Miscellaneous.

Major strokes

Most patients with cerebrovascular disease are first seen with a major stroke. There is usually a history of hypertension or TIAs. Cerebral thrombosis presents suddenly in over 50% of cases. Consciousness is often impaired and there is deviation of the head and eyes towards the side of the affected hemisphere. Initially, there is flaccid hemiparesis, becoming spastic with time. On the affected side the tendon jerks are brisk and the plantar response is extensor.

Cerebral infarction

Clinical distinction between cerebral infarction and haemorrhage is difficult. The patient presents with signs of rapid-onset hemiplegia, clouding of consciousness and frequently dysphasia. A bruit is sometimes heard over the carotid artery. The blood pressure may be elevated as a result of previous hypertension or cerebral oedema. Clinical examination may reveal the source of emboli, e.g. mitral stenosis with atrial fibrillation, bacterial endocarditis or recent myocardial infarction. Severe headache in the elderly patient should alert one to the possibility of temporal arteritis. Frequently,

patients present in deep coma, and death results from bronchopneumonia or from pulmonary embolism.

Cerebral haemorrhage

This occurs with sudden onset of severe headache, vomiting and unconsciousness. It is precipitated by physical exertion. In many cases there are signs of meningism and periodic breathing. Patients may have a history of high blood pressure with evidence of left ventricular failure. Intracerebral haemorrhage frequently involves the internal capsule, giving rise to a dense hemiplegia and hemianaesthesia.

Syndromes of the cerebral arteries

Internal carotid artery occlusion. This causes contralateral hemiplegia, facial palsy, hemianopia, hemianaesthesia and urinary incontinence. Furthermore, infarction of the dominant left hemisphere will result in dysphasia, which is usually of mixed type. Some patients may develop confusion. Infarction of the non-dominant right hemisphere produces severe perceptual problems, which can cause difficulty, particularly in elderly patients, as they may be incorrectly labelled as demented. There is also neglect of the left side of space, such as leaving half a plateful of food uneaten. Unilateral neglect may affect the patient's ability to draw and copy pictures.

Middle cerebral artery. This artery is commonly involved in cerebral thromboembolism. Occlusion will result in contralateral hemiplegia, sensory loss, motor aphasia and hemianopia.

Anterior cerebral artery. Occlusion of this vessel will cause contralateral hemiplegia with greater weakness of leg than arm, cortical sensory loss, aphasia and apraxia. The arm may show involuntary movements. Incontinence of urine and self-neglect may be additional problems.

Posterior cerebral artery. Involvement of the posterior cerebral artery produces contralateral homonymous hemianopia, contralateral thalamic syndrome and, if the visual association area in the dominant hemisphere is affected, there will be visual agnosia. Bilateral lesions of occipital lobes will cause total blindness of cortical type. The pupillary reflexes are normal. Frequently there is loss of memory and confusion. The mortality rate is high.

Vertebrobasilar territory syndromes. Total occlusion of the basilar artery is immediately fatal. Smaller infarcts will impair respiration, heart beat and level of consciousness. Involvement of the lower brain stem causes paralysis and sensory impairment in all limbs, and dysphagia. Lesions higher in the brain stem present with vertigo, vomiting, dysarthria, dysphagia and cerebellar signs. Occlusion of individual branches of the basilar artery can produce crossed hemiplegias. These are:

- *Weber's syndrome* — unilateral 3rd cranial nerve palsy with contralateral hemiplegia.
- *Benedikt's syndrome* — 3rd nerve palsy with ipsilateral cerebellar ataxia.
- *Millard–Gubler syndrome* — paralysis of 6th and 7th cranial nerves on one side with contralateral hemiplegia.
- *Foville's syndrome* — 6th nerve palsy, paralysis of conjugate ocular deviation and contralateral hemiplegia.

Vertebrobasilar ischaemia is common in the elderly and can cause symptoms of loss of balance, poor posture control, dizziness, recurrent falls and drop attacks.

Posterior inferior cerebellar artery. Occlusion of this branch of the vertebral artery gives a typical clinical picture. It consists of vertigo, vomiting, unilateral facial pain, dysphagia, paralysis of the palate on the side of the lesion, cerebellar signs in the limbs on the affected side, ipsilateral Horner's syndrome, dissociated anaesthesia to pain and temperature on the same side of the face and over the opposite half of the body below the neck.

Subarachnoid haemorrhage

The patient is usually aged between 30 and 60 years, and may have hypertension. In 60% of cases the source of haemorrhage is a ruptured aneurysm. There is sudden onset, with severe headache. Rapid loss of consciousness may occur, ending in coma and death. Often there are convulsions. Vomiting, meningism and confusion may occur. Bleeding around the aneurysm may compress the cranial nerves giving rise to focal signs, such as diplopia. An aneurysm may bleed into the brain, in which case the features are indistinguishable from cerebral haemorrhage. Examination of the fundus may show subhyaloid haemorrhage. Lumbar puncture will confirm the diagnosis and an angiogram or CT scan will show an aneurysm.

Minor strokes

Minor strokes are a form of TIA in which the symptoms persist for longer than 24 hours. They are also called 'reversible ischaemic neurological deficits'. Recurrent mini-strokes can lead to multi-infarct dementia.

Stroke-in-evolution

Here, the stroke develops gradually over a period of several hours, usually as a result of cerebral infarction. Cerebral tumours and subdural haematomas may present with a similar picture. An accurate diagnosis is essential, as there may be a chance of surgical intervention. An angiogram or CT scan will be required.

Transient ischaemic attacks (TIAs)

TIAs are acute, transient episodes of focal neurological or retinal dysfunction lasting less than 24 hours. Usually the deficit lasts only a few minutes. About 40% of these patients go on to develop a hemiplegic stroke within 2 years. TIAs are most frequently caused by micro-emboli arising from the heart or carotid artery and lodging in the small cerebral blood vessels. The resultant neuronal ischaemia is temporary, as the embolus breaks up and disperses. The micro-emboli consist of platelets, cholesterol and small amounts of fibrin. They form at the site of atheroma in the large neck vessels and from time to time break off and are carried up into the cerebral circulation. A carotid bruit is often heard.

Causes of TIAs

- Embolism of thrombotic material from necrotic atheromatous plaques in the neck arteries.
- Embolism from cardiac lesions.
- Transient cardiac arrhythmias.

Precipitating causes of TIAs

1 Cardiac disorders:

Tachycardias.

Heart block.

Low cardiac output.

Sick sinus syndrome.

Cardiac infarction.

Valvular disease.

2 Haematological disorders:

Polycythaemia.

Anaemia.

Diabetes.

Arteritis.

3 Blood pressure:

   Hypertension.

   Postural hypotension.

4 Vertebrobasilar atheroma plus cervical spine arthritis.

Clinical features of TIAs

A patient is rarely seen by the doctor at the time of the TIA, therefore diagnosis is made on the history and description of the symptoms. There are two main types: carotid TIAs — in the territory of the internal carotid artery; and vertebrobasilar TIAs — in the territory of the vertebrobasilar arteries. Their clinical features are as follows:

- Carotid TIAs:

   Amaurosis fugax — transient monocular blindness.

   Hemiparesis or monoparesis.

   Episodic confusion.

   Unilateral sensory disturbance.

   Dysphasia.

   Hemianopia.

- Vertebrobasilar TIAs:

   Visual disturbances — diplopia, hemianopia, cortical blindness.

   Vertigo.

   Dysarthria.

   Dysphasia.

   Circumoral paraesthesiae.

   Hemiparesis and sensory disturbances.

   Drop attacks.

   Memory loss.

Subclavian steal syndrome

Transient neurological symptoms occur in patients who have stenosis of the subclavian artery proximal to the origin of the vertebral artery. When the arm is exercised the blood flows in a retrograde direction down the vertebral artery resulting in symptoms of vertebrobasilar ischaemia. A bruit may be heard over the subclavian artery and there is a difference in blood pressure between the two arms.

Multiple infarct dementia

Small cerebral infarcts occurring with hypertension can lead to dementia in old age. The patient, usually an elderly man, suffers step-wise deterioration of both physical and mental health. Clinical features include weakness, slowness, depression, dysarthria, dysphagia, small-stepped gait, brisk tendon jerks and rigid limbs. Pseudobulbar palsy may develop. Memory begins to fail, and there is pathological laughing and weeping. Self-neglect, perseveration, incontinence, paranoid symptoms and immobility appear over a period of time. Sometimes the picture is very similar to advanced parkinsonism.

Boundary zone infarction

This occurs as a result of sudden hypotension. Ischaemia affects the boundary zones of the brain tissue between major arterial territories. The clinical picture depends upon the site of infarction.

Intracranial thrombophlebitis and cerebral venous thrombosis

Suppurative thrombophlebitis of the intracranial venous sinuses often affects the lateral cavernous and superior longitudinal sinuses as a result of spread of infection from the ear, face or frontal sinuses. Patients are acutely ill with high fever, headache and pyaemia.

Aseptic thrombosis of the cavernous sinus gives rise to the syndrome of benign intracranial hypertension, with headache and papilloedema. Cortical vein or dural sinus thrombosis may result in haemorrhagic cerebral infarction. Causes include dehydration, hyperviscosity, pregnancy and coagulation disorders.

Unruptured aneurysms

Unruptured aneurysms of cerebral vessels may give rise to symptoms and signs similar to those of an intracerebral space-occupying lesion.

Arteriovenous malformations

When these rupture they give rise to subarachnoid haemorrhage. Sometimes the patient may have focal fits, headache and varying neurological signs as the angioma expands.

Cerebellar haemorrhage

This is an unusual cause of stroke. It occurs suddenly with posterior headache, deteriorating consciousness, unilateral cerebellar signs, gaze palsy and sometimes medullary coning. It is important to diagnose this condition, as surgical evacuation of the haematoma may be possible.

Miscellaneous

Buerger's disease. This consists of thromboangiitis obliterans involving the cerebral blood vessels. The patient has fits, progressive dementia and variable palsies of the limbs.

Sturge–Weber syndrome. This is a congenital malformation of the precapillaries in the cerebral cortex involving usually one hemisphere and giving rise to a characteristic radiological pattern of subcortical calcification outlining the cerebral gyri.

Patients have fits, contralateral hemiparesis and a port wine naevus of the face on the affected side.

Pulseless disease (Takayasu's disease). This is a non-specific arteritis of the aortic arch that occurs in young people and results in slow progressive occlusion of the medium-sized arteries. Repeated cerebral infarctions occur, producing a variety of signs and symptoms.

Moya-Moya disease. This unusual disorder occurs mainly in people of Japanese origin. The pathology consists of multiple progressive intracranial arterial occlusions occurring in young adults, who may present with paralysis, fits, visual disorders, psychiatric symptoms and sometimes intracranial haemorrhage.

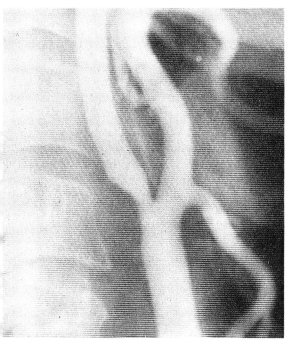

76 Angiogram showing stenosis at the origin of the internal carotid artery by atheromatous plaque; the patient presented with features of carotid TIAs.

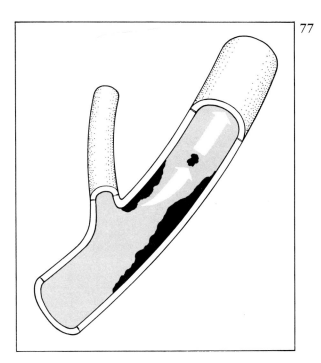

77

77 Atherosclerotic debris being shed from an atheromatous ulcer and entering the cerebral circulation, causing a transient ischaemic attack.

78 a), b), c), d), e), f), g) and h) Scanning electron microscope pictures of red blood corpuscles and platelets with pseudopodia in different stages of activity showing early steps in the formation of thrombus and platelet microemboli.

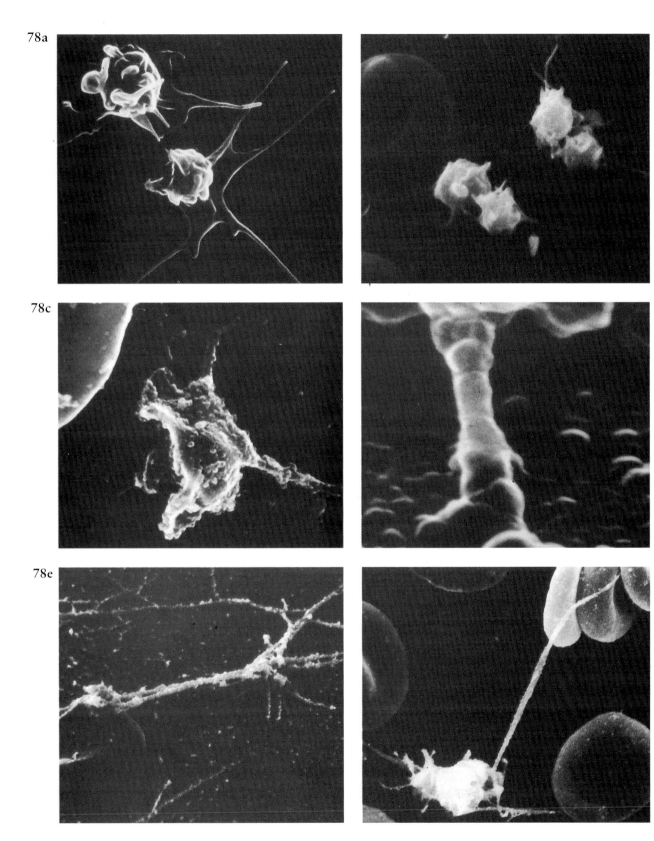

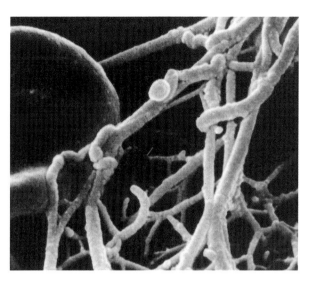
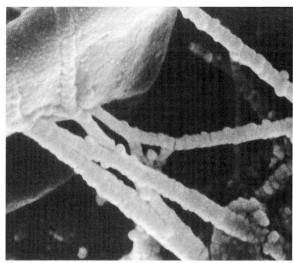

79 Scanning electron microscope picture of a small thrombus.

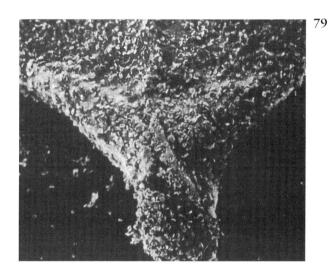

80 Recent platelet embolus in a small cerebral artery.

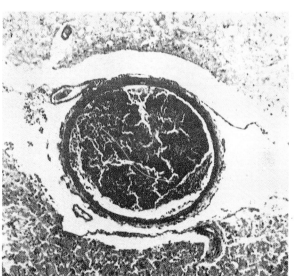

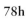

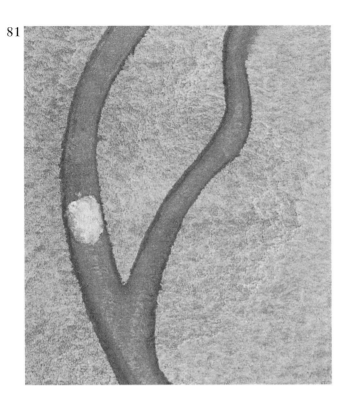

81

81 Ophthalmoscopic appearance of a small embolus seen as a refractile body filling the lumen of a branch of the retinal artery. This causes transient loss of vision (amaurosis fugax).

82

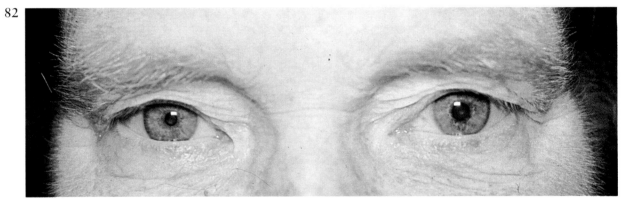

82 Unequal pupils in a case of intracerebral haemorrhage.

83

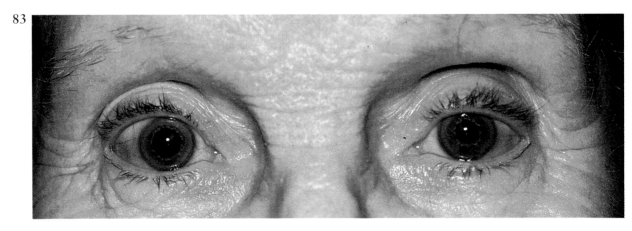

83 Unequal pupils in a case of subdural haematoma.

84 Recent hemiplegia. The eyes are deviated towards the side of the lesion.

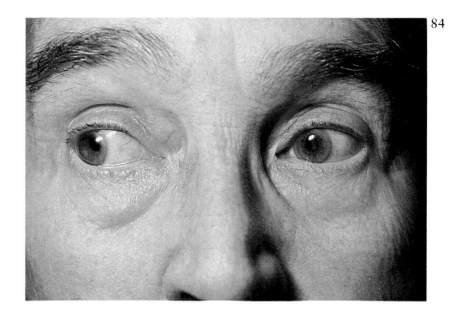

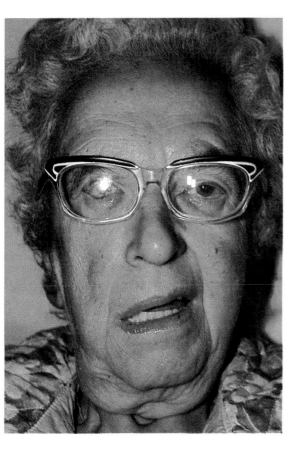

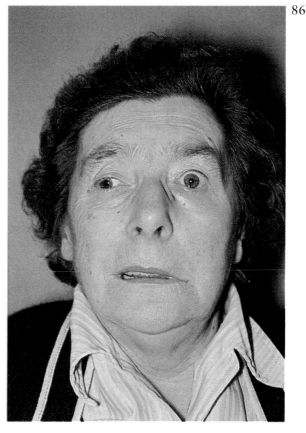

85 Right-sided facial palsy. The patient had right hemiplegia and complete aphasia.

86 Left-sided facial palsy. The patient also had perceptual problems.

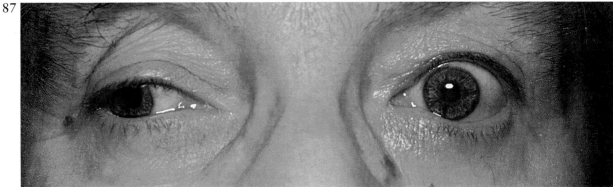

87 **Right-sided 3rd cranial nerve palsy** caused by a cerebrovascular lesion in a patient with diabetes mellitus. Note that the right eye is deviated laterally.

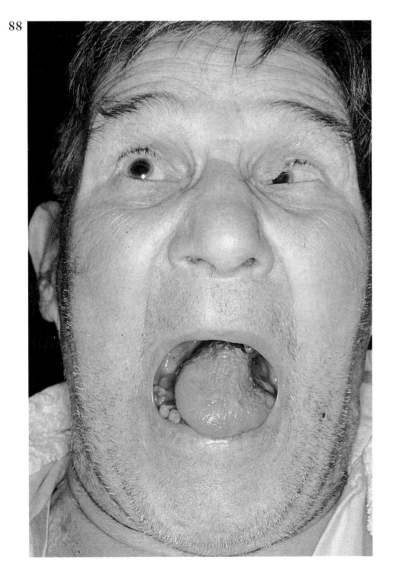

88 **Left-sided 6th and 12th cranial nerve palsies** in a patient who had recurrent strokes and clinical features of multi-infarct dementia. The left eye is deviated medially and there is paralysis of the left half of the tongue.

89 An elderly man with Horner's syndrome showing ptosis on the left side.

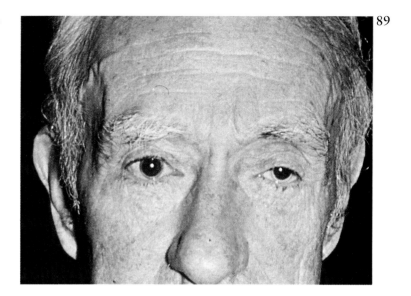

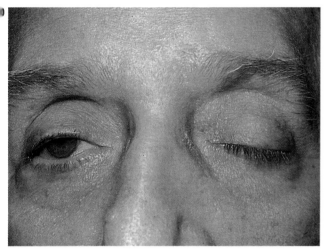

90 Left-sided ptosis caused by a lesion involving the cervical sympathetic chain.

91 Hemianopia. Diagram showing the changes in the field of vision produced by lesions at various points along the optic pathways. Homonymous hemianopia is the commonest defect produced with a hemiplegic stroke.

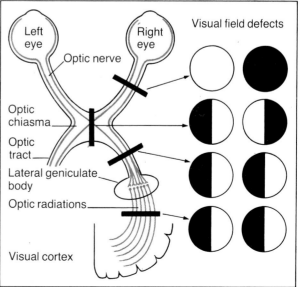

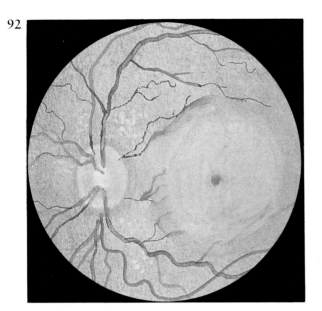

92 **Ophthalmoscopic view of central retinal artery thrombosis.** Artist's impression. Note the pallor resulting from ischaemia, and the 'cherry-red spot'.

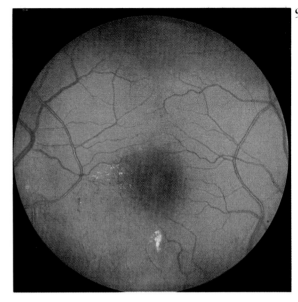

93 **Hypertensive fundus** with macular exudates.

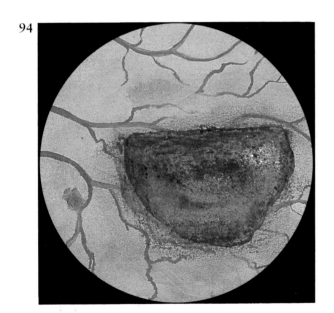

94 **Subhyaloid haemorrhage** in a case of subarachnoid haemorrhage. Artist's impression. Note the large half-moon shaped haemorrhage.

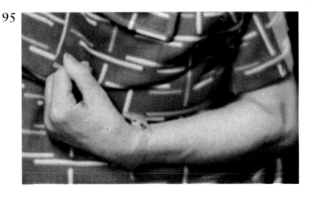

95 Spasticity of the hemiplegic left arm and hand.

96 Spasticity of the hemiplegic right hand.

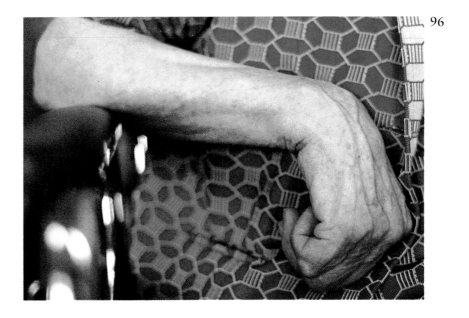

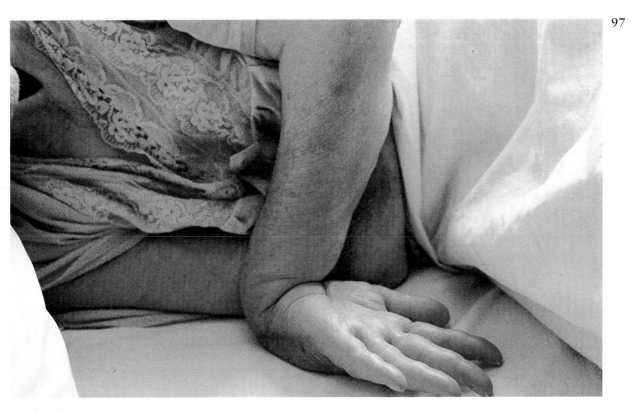

97 Flaccid paralysis of the arm.

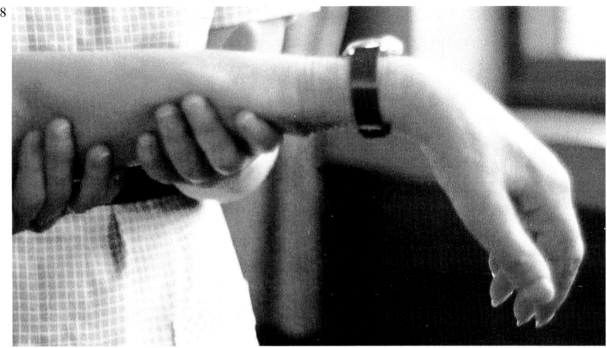

98 Wrist drop resulting from radial nerve palsy in a patient with monoplegia.

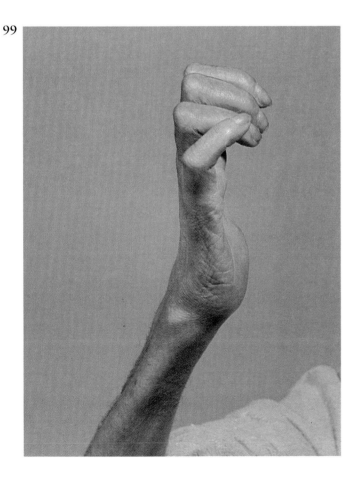

99 Wasting of the small muscles of the hand with 'claw-hand' deformity caused by ulnar nerve palsy.

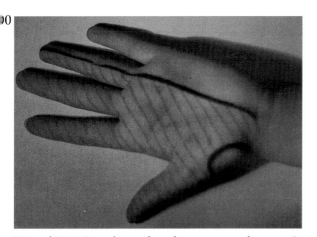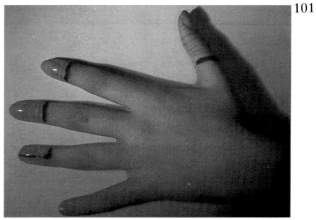

100 and **101 Carpal tunnel syndrome:** areas of sensory impairment as a result of a median nerve lesion. Carpal tunnel syndrome can occur in elderly stroke patients during the process of rehabilitation.

102 Hemiplegic oedema of the right hand; the patient also had right shoulder–hand syndrome.

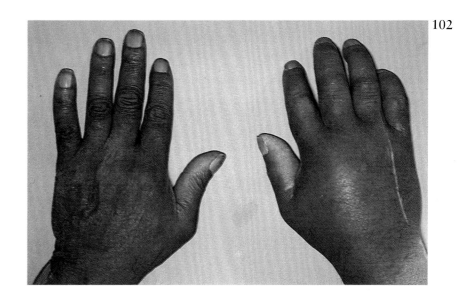

103 Hemiplegic oedema of the left arm.

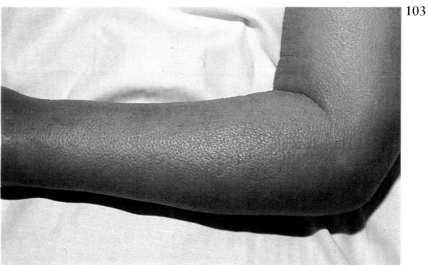

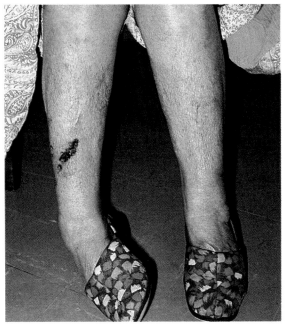

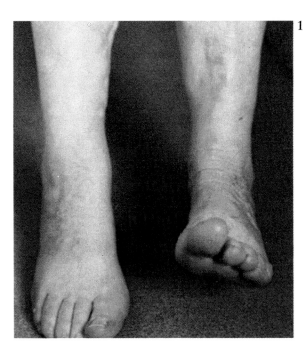

104 Hemiplegic posture of the right leg. The patient should practise keeping both feet squarely on the floor.

105 Foot drop in a case of right hemiplegia.

106 Foot drop caused by peroneal nerve palsy as a result of prolonged pressure over the head of the fibula.

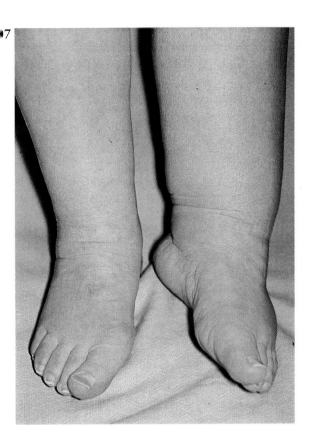

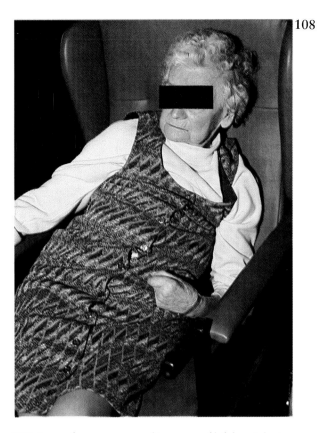

107 Hemiplegic oedema of the left foot. Diuretics are of little benefit but physiotherapy, mobilisation and limb elevation should improve the condition.

108 Loss of posture control in a case of left hemiplegia. The patient ignored the left half of her body space and had perceptual problems.

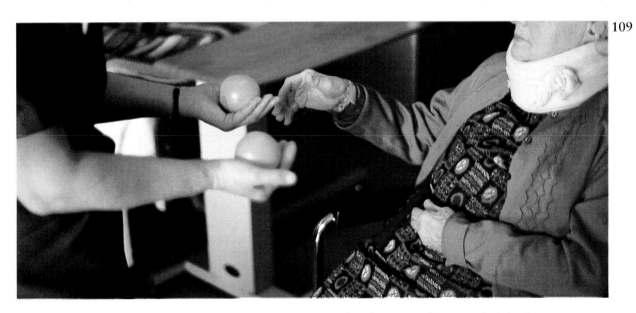

109 Left-sided neglect. The patient is presented with two oranges but she ignores the one on the left side.

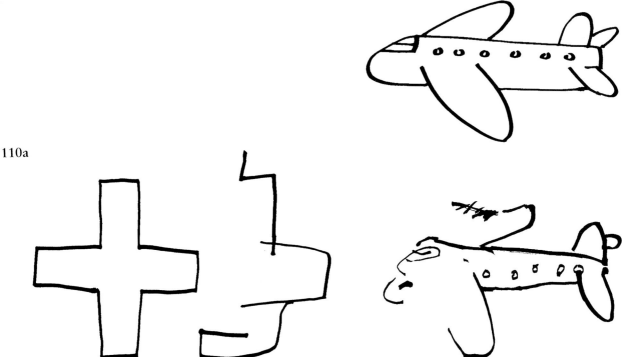

110a

110 a) and b) This patient had a right cerebral infarction and mild left hemiparesis. He was asked to copy figures of a cross and an aeroplane. In each drawing he has ignored the left side of the picture without realising his error because of left-sided neglect.

111

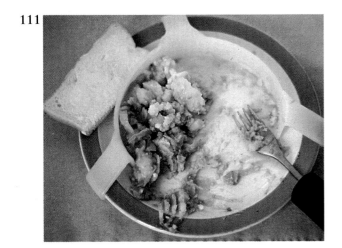

111 Unilateral neglect. The patient has left the food uneaten on the left half of the plate.

11

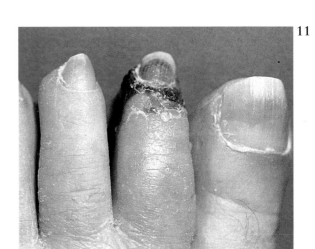

112 Peripheral vascular disease often coexists in elderly patients who have suffered a stroke. Full clinical examination will reveal features of widespread atheroma.

113 Raynaud's phenomenon resulting from systemic lupus erythematosus. The patient had also suffered a minor stroke.

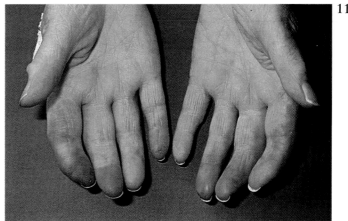

114 Plethoric face of a patient with polycythaemia. He presented with features of cardiac failure and transient ischaemic attacks.

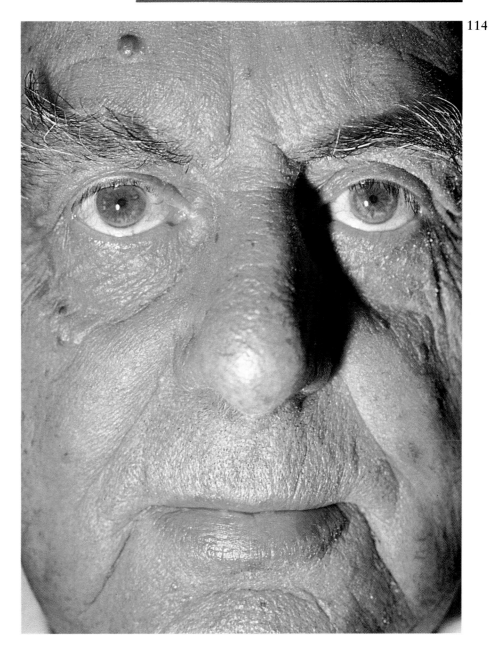

115a

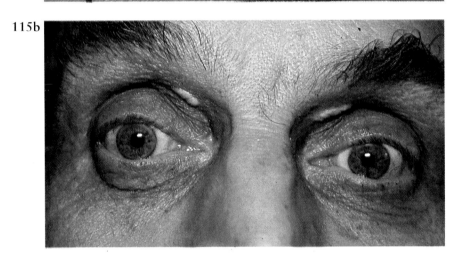

115b

115 a) and b) Xanthelasma in a patient who presented with ischaemic heart disease and had a family history of hyperlipidaemia and strokes.

116

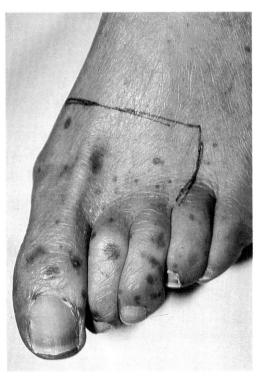

116 Subacute bacterial endocarditis showing small embolic infarcts on the toes. Patients can develop cerebral embolism.

117 Opened heart showing
vegetations of bacterial
endocarditis on the valvular rim.

117

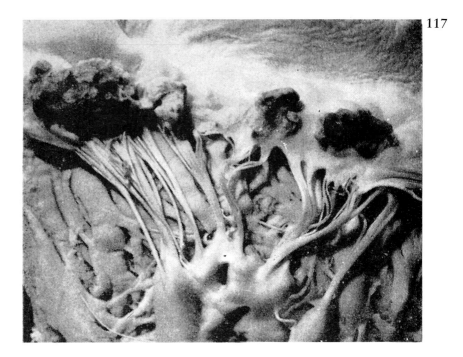

118 Polyarteritis nodosa. Severe
vasculitis resulting in ischaemic
necrosis of the toes. Some patients
go on to develop cerebral
infarction.

118

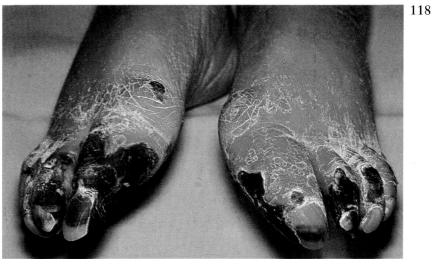

119 Severe vasculitis in a case of
polyarteritis nodosa. The patient
had arthralgia, hypertension,
renal failure and a minor stroke.

119

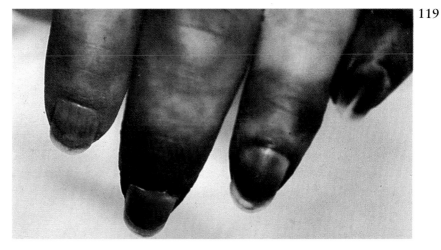

120

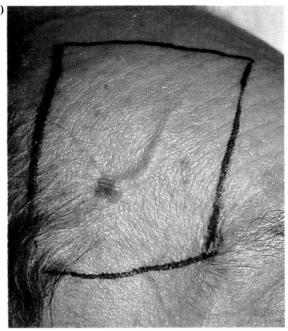

120 Temporal arteritis. Urgent treatment with corticosteroids is required if blindness and cerebral infarction are to be avoided.

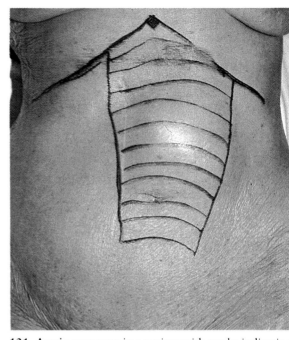

121 Aortic aneurysm in a patient with stroke indicating generalised atheroma.

122

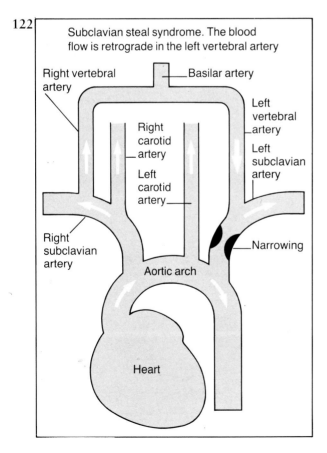

Subclavian steal syndrome. The blood flow is retrograde in the left vertebral artery

Right vertebral artery

Basilar artery

Left vertebral artery

Right carotid artery

Left subclavian artery

Left carotid artery

Right subclavian artery

Narrowing

Aortic arch

Heart

122 Diagrammatic representation of the mechanism of 'subclavian steal' syndrome. Patients with this condition usually present with black-outs or other transient neurological symptoms.

123 Boundary zone infarction. Ischaemia (yellow) affects the boundary zones between major arterial territories.

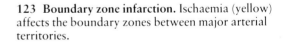
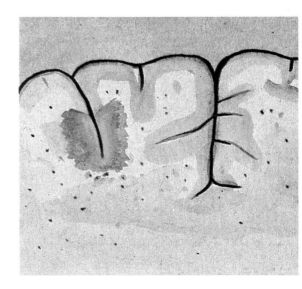

124 Multi-infarct dementia.
This patient had suffered
several strokes and both mental
and physical states showed
stepwise deterioration.

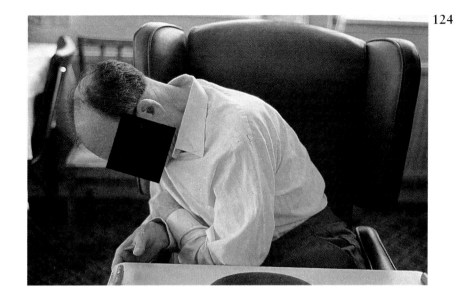

**125 Primitive reflexes are
positive in disease of the frontal
lobes** — particularly senile and
multi-infarct dementia. In the
grasp reflex pressure applied
by the examiner's fingertips
moving towards the patient's
fingertips on the flexor tendons
causes a grasp.

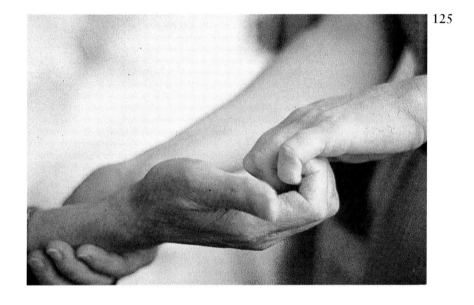

126 Sturge–Weber syndrome. The patient
had fits, contralateral hemiparesis and a
port wine naevus of the face on the affected
side.

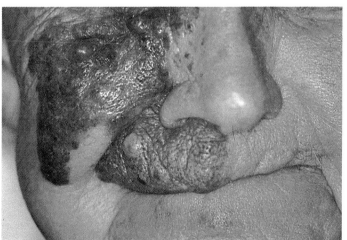

DIFFERENTIAL DIAGNOSIS

A typical stroke occurs with sudden onset in a known hypertensive and causes focal neurological signs, usually hemiplegia and drowsiness. In such cases the diagnosis of cerebral infarction is straightforward. However, occasionally, confusion may arise, particularly in elderly patients where an accurate history may not be available and the clinical picture is atypical. In such cases other possibilities must be considered, as very often they present with a 'stroke-like' syndrome.

Subdural haematoma. This can easily be missed, especially in elderly patients. The symptoms and signs may fluctuate but the patient deteriorates slowly. A cranial echogram will show shift of midline structures and a brain scan will confirm the diagnosis.

Brain tumours. Both primary and secondary cerebral tumours (gliomas, meningiomas, metastases from carcinoma of the lung) can present with a stroke-like illness, especially if the tumour expands rapidly or if there is associated bleeding. About 5% of patients presenting with a stroke have an intracranial tumour.

Acute infections, e.g. meningitis, encephalitis, abscess. Infections involving the brain may present with focal features suggestive of a stroke. The patient is drowsy and has features of meningism and fever. The CSF shows typical abnormalities. In some, the picture may be further complicated by secondary arteritis and thrombosis.

Hypertensive encephalopathy. The patient has headaches, vomiting, fits, confusion and focal neurological signs. Diastolic blood pressure is above 130 mm Hg and there may be papilloedema. Signs subside with lowering of the blood pressure.

Epilepsy. This can cause diagnostic difficulties if the patient presents with coma and witnesses are not available. Unilateral paralysis may persist for several hours after a fit (Todd's paralysis). A past history of convulsions should clarify the picture.

Metabolic disorders. Several metabolic abnormalities, especially of acute onset, can present with a stroke-like picture, e.g. hypoglycaemia, uraemia, myxoedema, hepatic failure.

Cerebellar haemorrhage. This presents with sudden severe occipital headache, vomiting and deteriorating level of consciousness. The pupils are constricted and there may be cerebellar signs. Prognosis is poor.

Drugs. Again, in the elderly, the effect of drugs can be confused with a stroke. The patient may have taken hypnotics with alcohol, resulting in coma.

Hypothermia. Patients with hypothermia are drowsy, lethargic and cold, with a temperature below 35°C. Hypothermia can cause cerebral thrombosis in elderly patients.

Acute systemic infections, e.g. septicaemia, cerebral malaria.

Migraine. This may present with a picture similar to mini-strokes or TIAs. Rarely, it gives rise to cerebral infarction.

Disseminated sclerosis. This may present with recurrent episodic neurological features, but detailed history and examination should clarify the diagnosis.

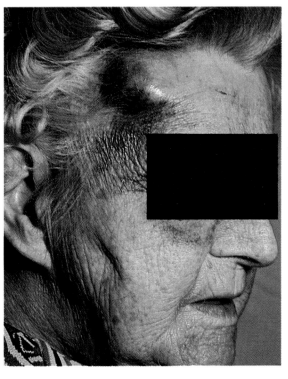

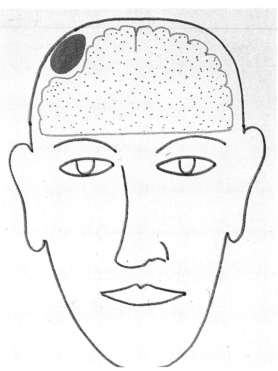

127 Head injury without underlying skull fracture.
This elderly patient subsequently developed confusion,
falls, vomiting and incontinence. An isotope scan
suggested subdural haematoma.

**128 Diagrammatic representation of subdural
haematoma.** Note the haematoma compressing the
brain tissue.

**129 Isotope scan of left-sided subdural
haematoma.**

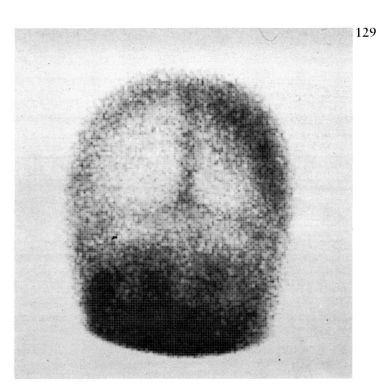

129

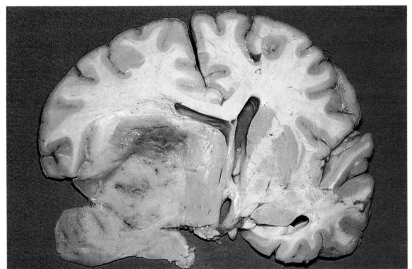

130 Section of brain showing an astrocytoma. The patient had died from a stroke-like illness.

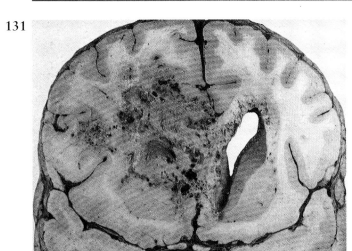

131 Section of brain showing glioblastoma multiforme with extensive infiltration and destruction of brain tissue. It has an ill-defined edge with regions of necrosis and cystic spaces.

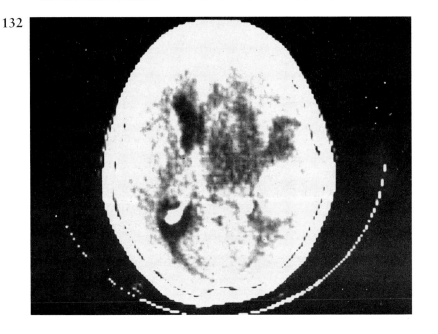

132 CT scan showing a right-sided glioma.

133 CT scan showing a left convexed meningioma. The patient had contralateral upper motor neurone signs.

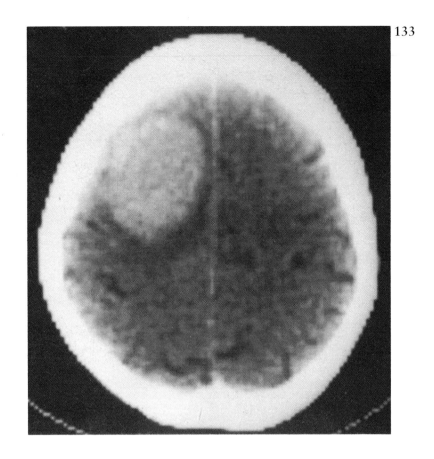

134 Isotope scan showing multiple metastases in a patient who was originally diagnosed as a case of multi-infarct dementia.

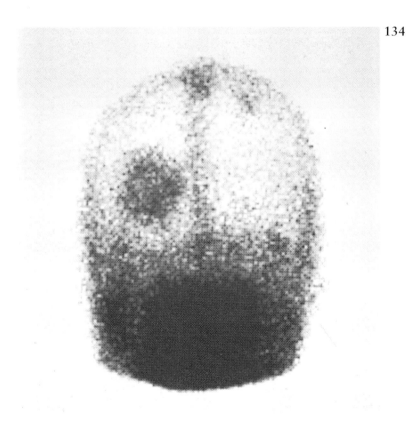

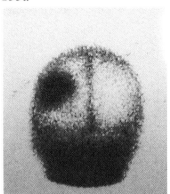
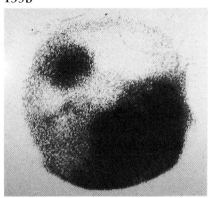

135 Isotope scan: a) posterior and b) lateral view of a large solitary brain tumour. The patient had signs of right hemiparesis.

136

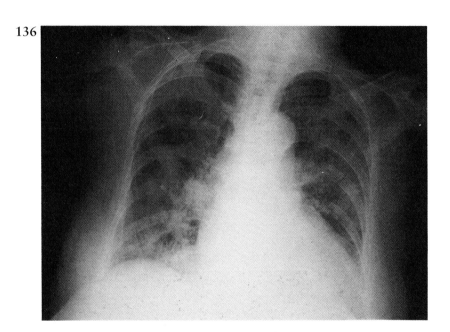

136 X-ray of the chest showing pulmonary metastases. The patient was admitted as an emergency with confusion and monoplegia. CT scan revealed cerebral secondaries.

137

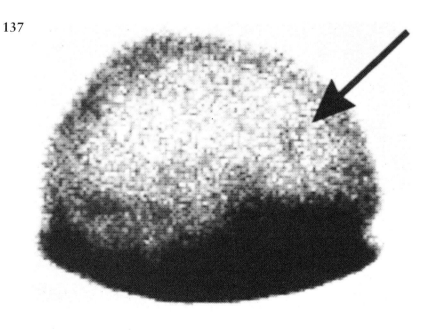

137 Isotope scan showing a single focus of increased uptake in the frontal region, a metastasis from a primary carcinoma of the lung.

138 CT scan showing multiple cerebral metastases.

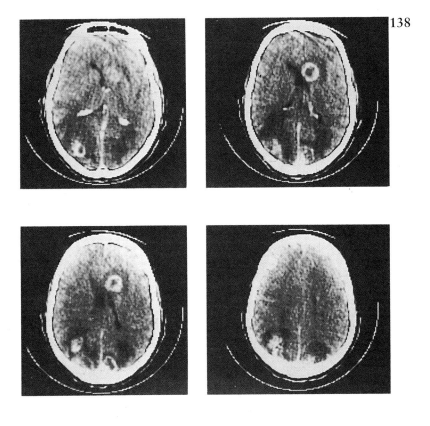

139 CT scan showing a cerebral **abscess** on the left of the corpus callosum, partly obliterating the body of the lateral ventricle.

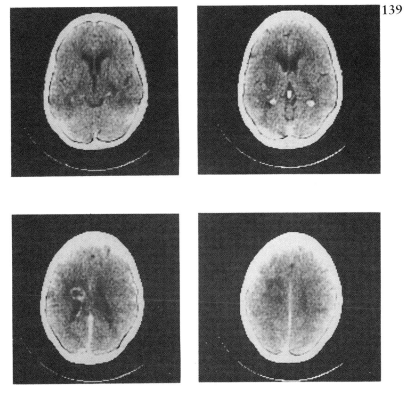

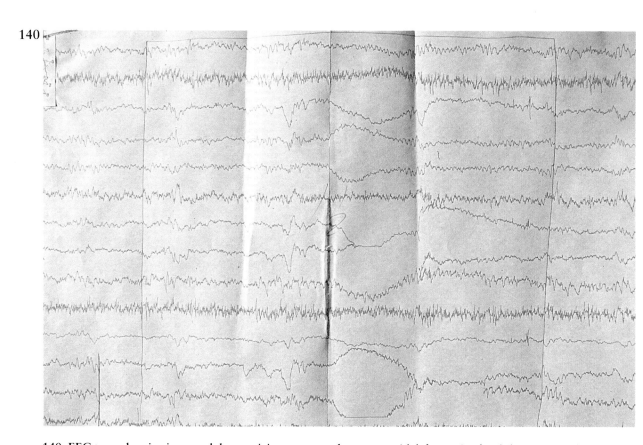

140 EEG trace showing increased theta activity as a general response with left anterior focal sharp wave. This patient had cortical epilepsy that presented with a 'stroke'.

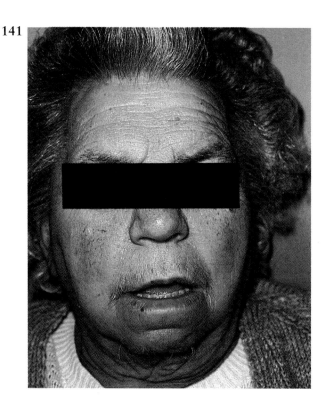

141 This elderly lady was admitted having collapsed, with provisional diagnosis of cerebral haemorrhage. Her body temperature was 31°C and she turned out to have underlying hypothyroidism.

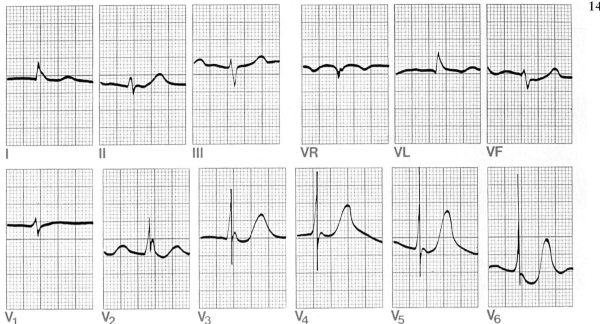

I II III VR VL VF

V₁ V₂ V₃ V₄ V₅ V₆

142 ECG from a patient with hypothermia, showing the typical J wave in V₂.

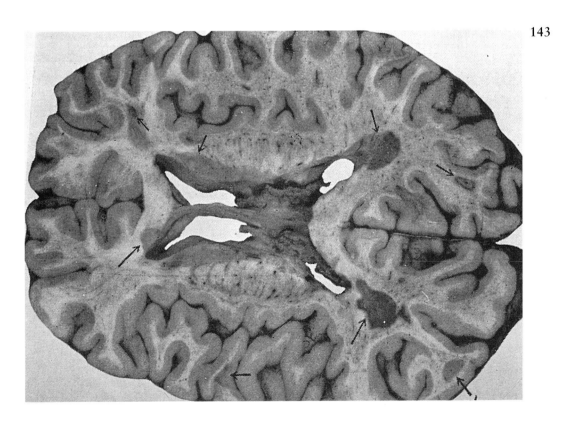

143 Horizontal section of brain from a patient with disseminated sclerosis. The arrows point to the numerous well-defined plaques.

INVESTIGATIONS

In cases where the aetiology of a stroke is obvious, further investigations are unnecessary. In elderly patients, 'stroke' is an acceptable diagnosis and it may be inappropriate to carry out complicated tests. However, TIAs and mini-strokes require a thorough work-up, especially in a young or middle-aged patient. Investigations are necessary to determine aetiological factors and to identify vascular abnormalities. The physician in charge will decide which investigations to perform, bearing in mind the past history, clinical examination and the age of the patient.

Blood tests

Full blood count. The patient may have anaemia or polycythaemia, Check the platelet count to exclude thrombocythaemia. The haematocrit may be raised, suggesting polycythaemia. Sickle cell disease and leukaemias may be discovered. A raised ESR may give a clue to temporal arteritis or multiple myeloma.

Blood sugar level. TIAs or minor strokes in a diabetic patient indicate atheroma with arterial damage.

Blood lipids. Hyperlipidaemia may be found in some younger patients with a family history of coronary artery disease or strokes.

Blood Wassermann reaction (VDRL test). Tests for syphilis should be done in an atypical case to avoid missing syphilitic arteritis.

Creatinine phosphokinase (CPK). This is raised after a recent myocardial infarction. A number of elderly patients who have had a myocardial infarction first present with a stroke. Mural thrombus can give rise to cerebral embolism. CPK is also elevated in the CSF following cerebral infarction.

Electrocardiogram (ECG)

This is done to detect a recent myocardial infarction, arrhythmia, hypertensive heart disease or cardiomyopathy. Twenty-four-hour ECG monitoring with computer-assisted analysis of the recorded tape is indicated if there is a possibility of transient cardiac arrhythmia (sick sinus syndrome or atrioventricular block with asystole) giving rise to a TIA or a minor stroke.

144

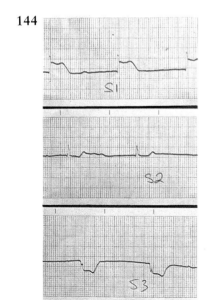 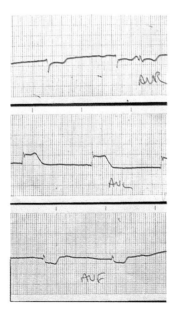

144 ECG showing a large myocardial infarction. There is ST elevation and T wave inversion. Mural thrombus can give rise to cerebral embolism. In elderly patients, hypotension can cause cerebral infarction.

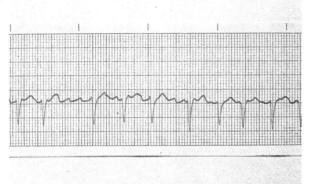

145 ECG showing fast atrial fibrillation — the patient was admitted with postural hypotension and repeated falls.

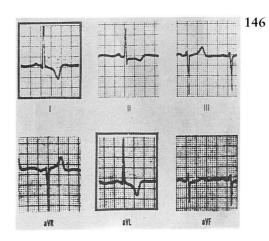

146 ECG showing left ventricular hypertrophy in a case of long-standing hypertension. Note ST depression and T wave inversion.

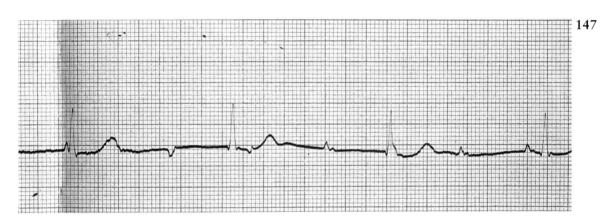

147 ECG showing complete heart block. The patient had suffered a number of minor strokes. Note that the ventricular complexes are completely independent of P waves.

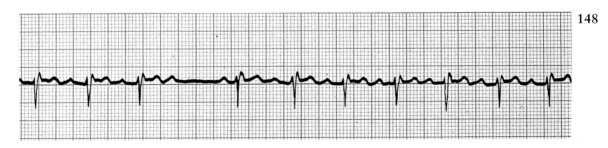

148 ECG showing Mobitz type II atrioventricular block with asystole. This can cause a serious fall in cerebral perfusion.

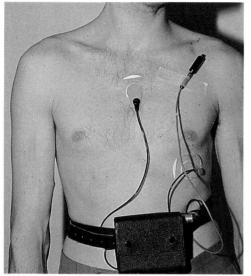

149 Twenty-four-hour ambulatory ECG being recorded on a portable machine.

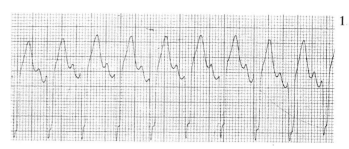

150a Transient cardiac arrhythmia shown up on a 24-hour ECG. The patient complained of fainting during this episode of tachycardia.

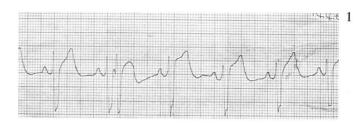

150b Twenty-four-hour ECG recording showing occasional atrial ectopic.

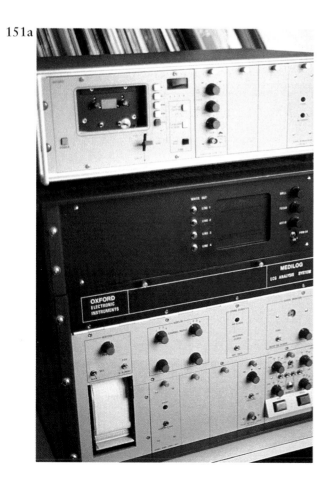

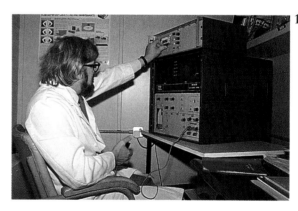

151 a) and b) Twenty-four-hour ECG tape being analysed on a playback computer system.

Echocardiography

This may show septal defects, valvular deformity, e.g. prolapsed mitral valve, or rarely atrial myxoma. Echocardiography is only rarely indicated in elderly patients.

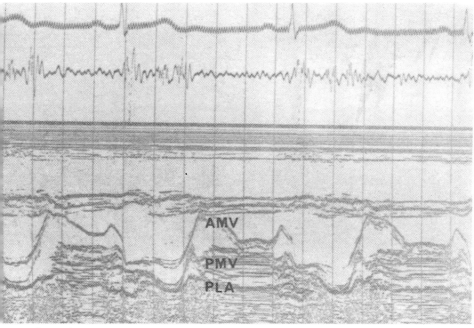

152

152 Echocardiogram of severe mitral valve prolapse. An apex phonocardiogram demonstrated the midsystolic click. AMV = anterior mitral leaflet motion; PMV = posterior mitral leaflet motion; PLA = posterior left atrial wall.

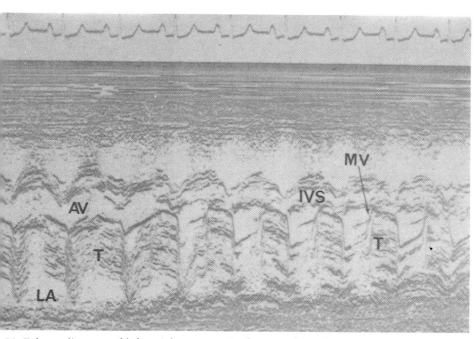

153

153 Echocardiogram of left atrial myxoma. In this scan from the aorta and the left atrium inferiorly to the mitral valve, the tumour was seen in the left atrium during systole, moving into the mitral orifice during diastole. AV = aortic valve motion; LA = left atrium; IVS = interventricular septum; MV = anterior mitral leaflet motion; T = tumour.

Electroencephalography (EEG)

This test is indicated if there is suspicion of focal epilepsy; its main benefit lies in differentiating between epilepsy and strokes. However, the record between the seizures may be negative. EEG cannot differentiate between cerebral infarction and a cerebral tumour.

154

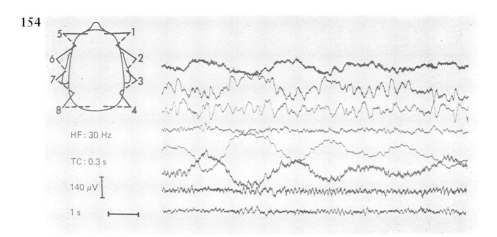

154 EEG 1 day after a massive right cerebral infarct. Note gross asymmetry of alpha rhythm, delta activity and sharp waves.

155

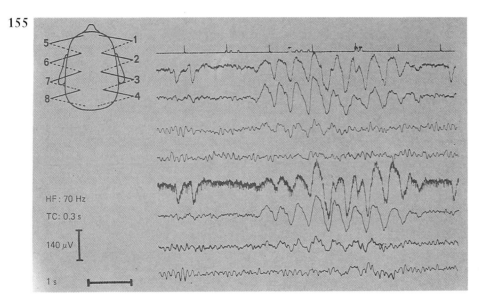

155 EEG of ruptured aneurysm of anterior communicating artery. There is frontal intermittent delta activity with anterior thalamic damage.

156

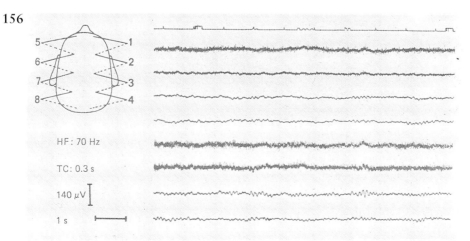

156 Asymmetrical EEG following occlusion of the right middle cerebral artery 1 month previously.

Aneurysm - localized dilation of a blood vessel

Radiology

Straight x-ray of the skull. This is rarely helpful but is indicated to rule out skull fracture in cases of head injury. Occasionally, brain tumours may show calcification or hyperostosis, and a shift of the pineal may be seen with intracerebral space-occupying lesions. Calcification in the carotid siphon indicates advanced atheroma.

X-ray of the chest. This may show increase in heart size caused by hypertension, mitral valve disease, unfolding of the aorta, aortic aneurysm, left ventricular aneurysm and cancer of the lung. All these conditions are associated with strokes.

X-ray of the cervical spine. In elderly patients there may be chronic degenerative changes in the cervical spine. Cervical spine disease may contribute to vertebrobasilar insufficiency and cause drop attacks.

157 Plain x-ray of the skull showing enlargement of the sella turcica. The patient had a pituitary tumour with visual field defects and acromegaly.

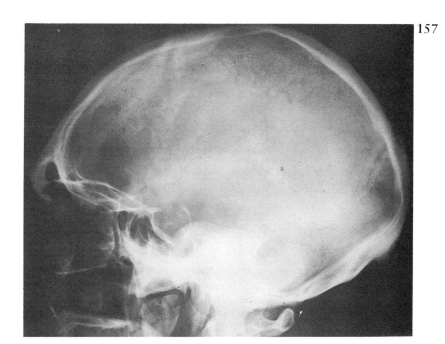

157

158 Plain x-ray of the skull showing hyperostosis secondary to a sphenoid wing meningioma.

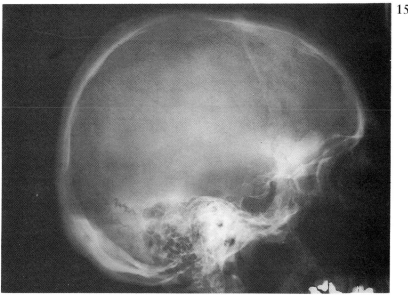

158

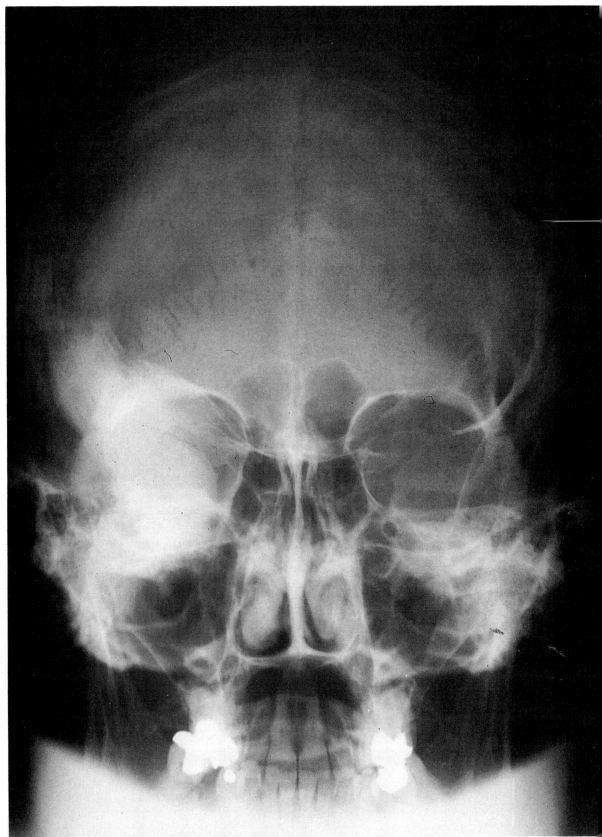

159 Plain x-ray of the skull, frontal view, showing hyperostosis secondary to a sphenoid wing meningioma.

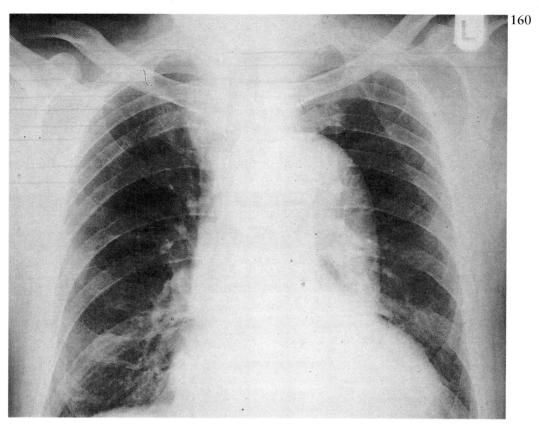

160 Plain x-ray of the chest showing unfolded aorta in an elderly patient with hypertension and stroke.

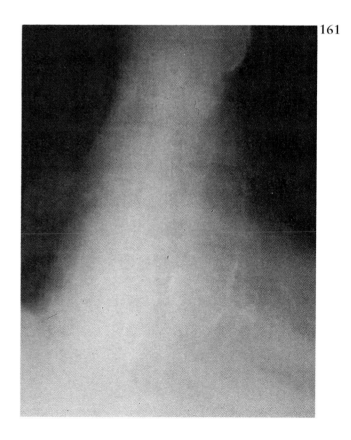

161 Plain x-ray of the chest showing calcification in the wall of an atheromatous aorta.

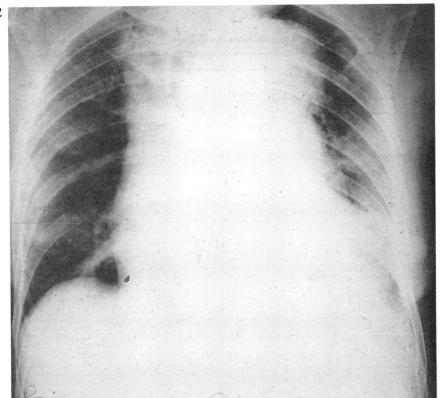

162 Plain x-ray of the chest showing a large aortic aneurysm. The patient had symptoms of TIAs.

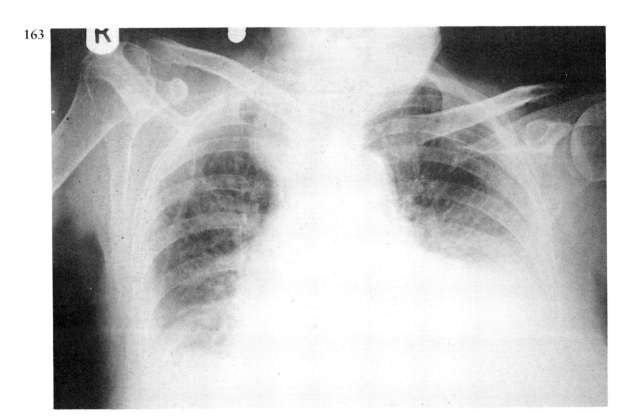

163 Plain x-ray of the chest in a patient with cerebral infarction and left ventricular failure.

164 Plain x-ray of the chest showing left ventricular aneurysm following a myocardial infarction. Such patients are at risk from cerebral embolism.

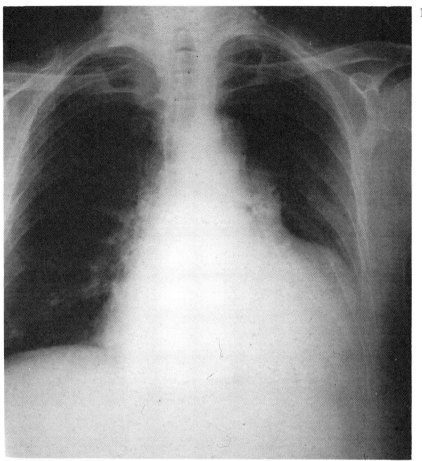

165 Plain x-ray of the chest showing a carcinoma in the right upper lobe of the lung. The patient presented with a stroke-like illness caused by cerebral metastases.

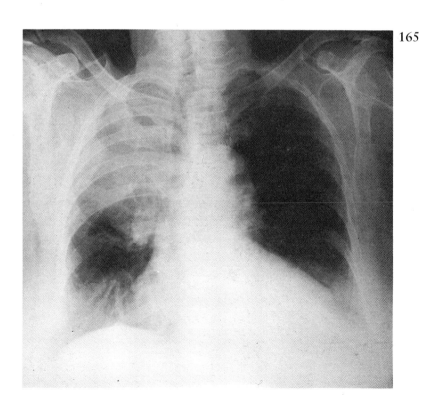

166

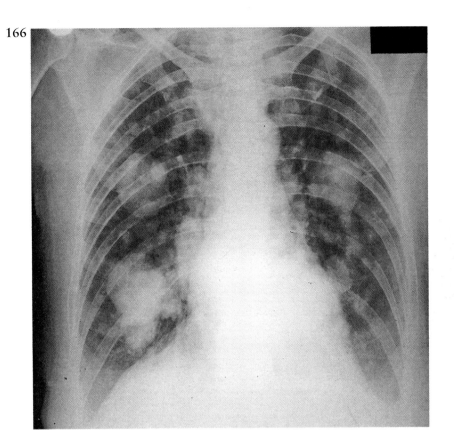

166 Plain x-ray of the chest showing pulmonary metastases from a malignant melanoma. The patient also had dysphasia caused by cerebral secondaries.

167

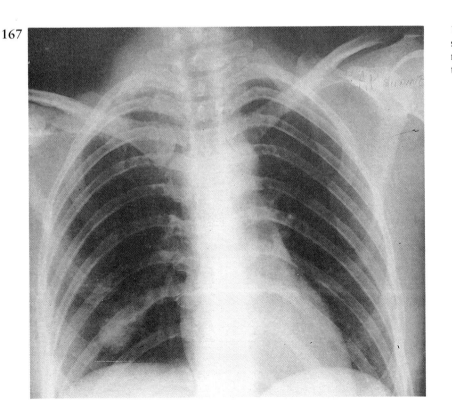

167 Plain x-ray of the chest showing arteriovenous malformation. This can give rise to cerebral embolism.

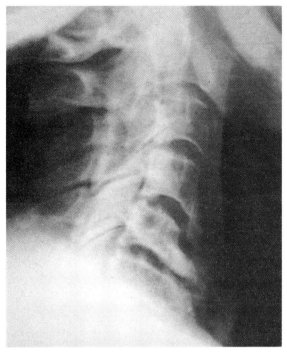

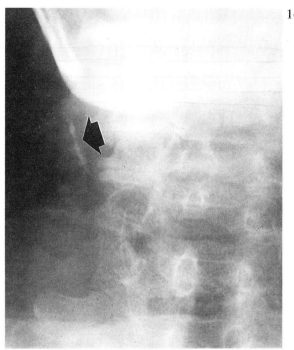

168 X-ray of the cervical spine showing cervical spondylosis. The patient suffered with drop attacks as a result of vertebrobasilar ischaemia.

169 Plain x-ray of the cervical spine showing calcification in the right carotid artery. This elderly patient complained of unsteadiness and falls.

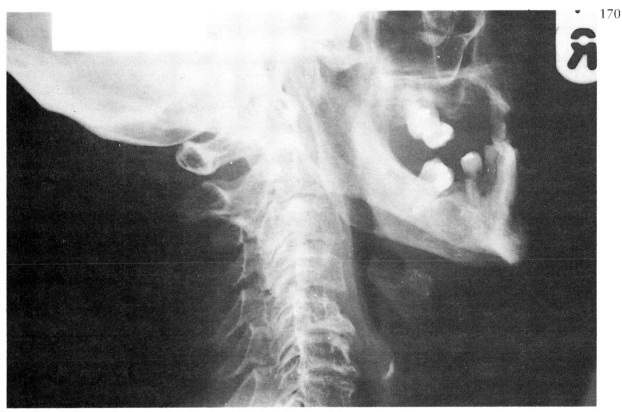

170 X-ray of the cervical spine showing deposits of myeloma and degenerative changes. The patient complained of unsteadiness, falls and vertigo.

Isotope brain scan

Synthetic radioisotope scanning is a useful preliminary to a CT scan. Where CT scanning is not available, a radioisotope scan can give useful information. The normal brain tissue does not take up any injected radioisotope and appears on the scan as a pale, 'cold' area. In cases of cerebral infarction the brain scan becomes positive within the first 7 days. Cerebral haemorrhage, cerebral tumours and subdural haematomas can be identified.

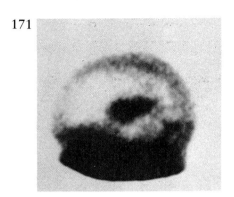

171 Isotope scan showing left middle cerebral artery infarct.

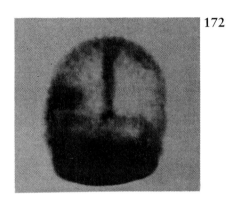

172 Isotope scan showing a large middle cerebral artery infarct.

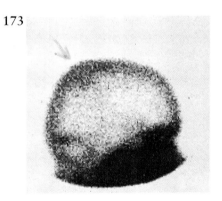

173 Recent cerebral infarct. The isotope scan shows a small area of diffusely increased activity in the right superior parietal region.

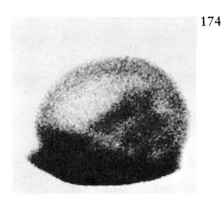

174 Isotope scan showing cerebral infarction. There is a large area of increased uptake in the parietal and occipital regions of the left hemisphere.

175

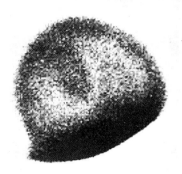

175 Isotope scan showing a recent cerebral infarction. A large wedge-shaped area of increased uptake can be seen in the right hemisphere.

176

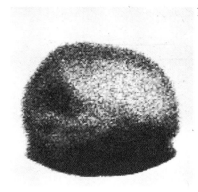

176 Isotope scan of a patient who had left hemiplegia, a visual field defect and neglect of left hemi-space. There is a large area of densely increased activity laterally in the right occipital region.

177

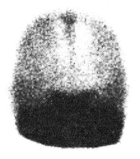

177 Isotope scan of a patient with dementia and pseudobulbar palsy. The scan shows widespread and patchy increase in activity in both hemispheres.

178

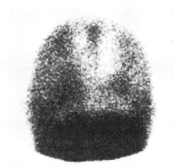

178 Isotope scan of a patient with long-standing dementia and bilateral upper motor neurone signs. The scan shows areas of multiple cerebral infarcts.

179

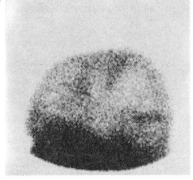

179 Isotope scan of a patient with multiple strokes. There are two distinct wedge-shaped areas superficially in the right posterior frontal region and parietal region.

180

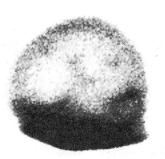

180 Isotope scan of a patient with dementia, hemiplegia and incontinence. The scan shows multiple focal areas of increased uptake.

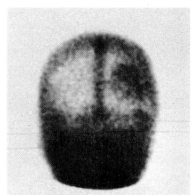

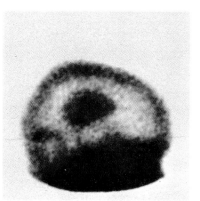

181 Isotope scans in a patient with a primary brain tumour. a) and **b)** show anterior and lateral cerebral views. The patient had headache, vomiting, confusion and dysphasia.

182

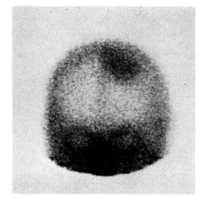

183

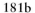

182 Isotope scan of a convexed meningioma causing stroke-like symptoms.

183 Isotope scan of a patient who presented with progressive dementia. Cerebral atrophy is just noticeable.

184a

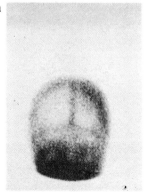

184b

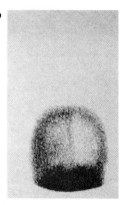

184 Isotope scan (anterior and posterior) showing left-sided subdural haematoma.

Cranial echogram

This is useful in cases of suspected subdural haematoma as it will reveal a shift of midline structures.

185 Cranial echogram showing a normal pattern.

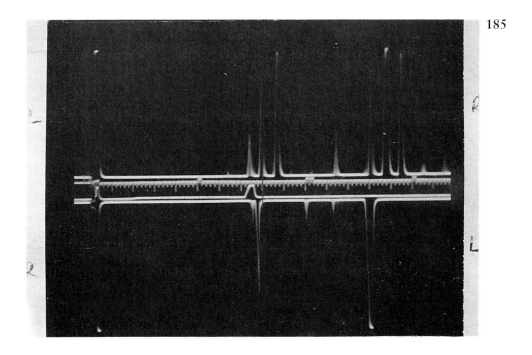

186 Cranial echogram showing a 5 mm shift to the left. The large upright deflection is shifted to the left, indicating compression from the right side. The patient had a right subdural haematoma.

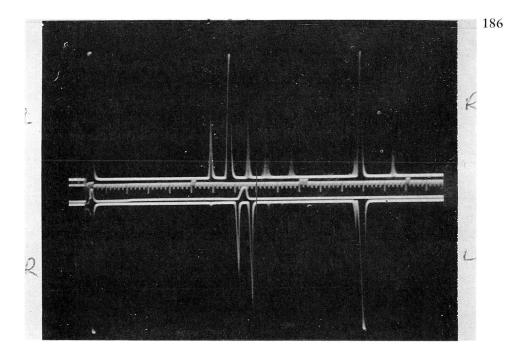

Computerised axial tomography (CT scanning)

The advent of CT scanning has meant that the pathology of strokes can be studied without recourse to invasive diagnostic tests. The principle of CT scanning draws on the technology of tomography and the differing absorption coefficients of the human tissues. Ideally, a CT scan should be done in every case of TIA or a minor stroke, but in practice this is rarely possible.

Indications for CT scanning in strokes

- A stroke presenting with atypical features.
- If there is doubt about the patient having had a stroke at all.
- To distinguish between stroke and tumour.
- To exclude intracranial haemorrhage in patients being considered for carotid endarterectomy.

- Spontaneous subarachnoid haemorrhage.
- In stroke that may be surgically treatable, e.g. supratentorial haematomas, cerebellar haematomas, arteriovenous malformations or aneurysms.
- In TIAs before angiography is considered.

Other indications for CT scanning are: raised intracranial pressure, cerebral abscess, head injury, encephalitis, coma of unknown cause, unexplained dementia, and epilepsy of late onset.

A CT scan in a patient with stroke may show infarction, haemorrhage, tumours, meningiomas, angiomas and metastases. Multiple small infarcts may be seen, even if the clinical examination is negative. Aneurysms both large and small are also shown.

187
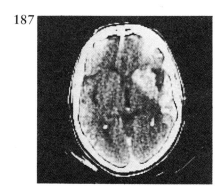 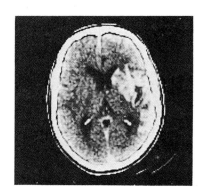
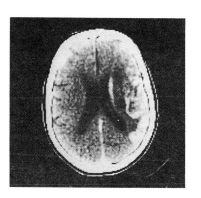 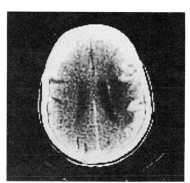

187 Enhance scans of recent right middle cerebral artery infarct.

188 CT scan of long-standing middle cerebral artery infarct.

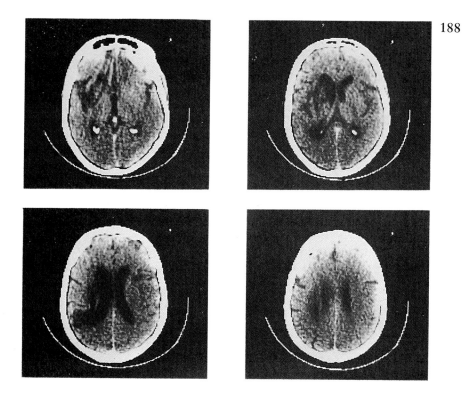

189 CT scan showing **symmetrical ventricular dilatation** with small focal areas of reduced attenuation in both parietal lobes — cerebrovascular disease with two areas of infarction.

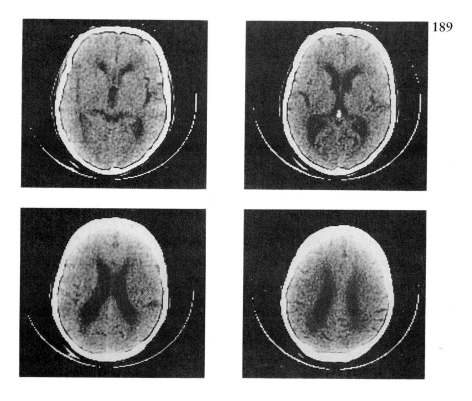

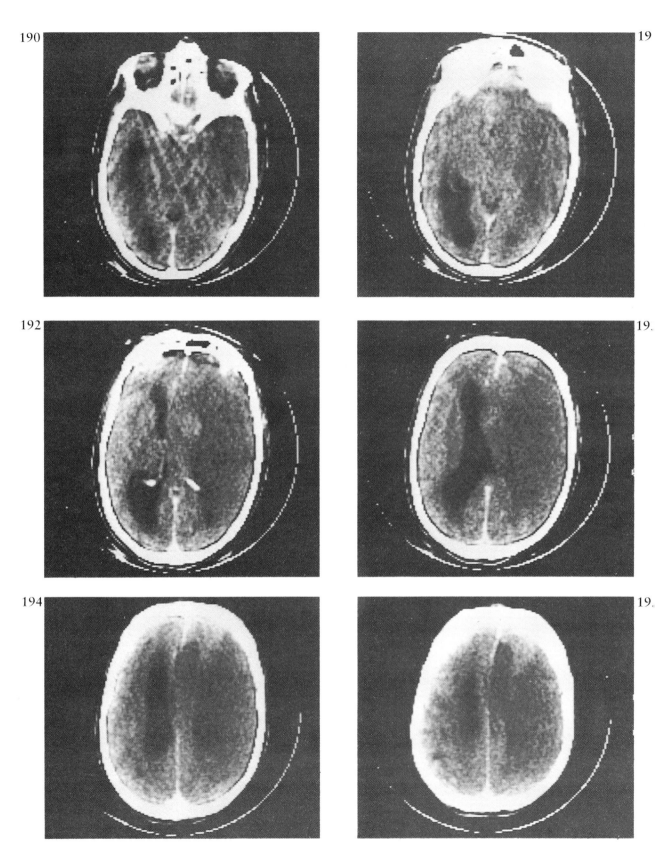

190–195 CT scans showing gross swelling of the right hemisphere caused by infarction of much of the hemisphere secondary to a carotid occlusion. There is dilatation of the contralateral ventricle as a result of swelling on the right side with obstruction to CSF flow.

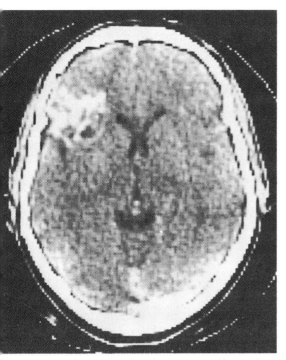 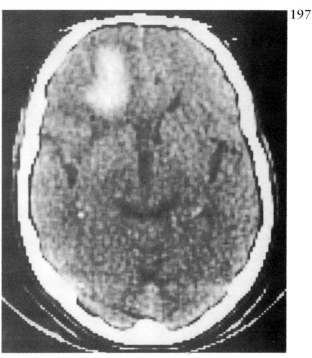

196 CT scan showing an arteriovenous malformation.

197 CT scan of a large mass in the left frontal lobe — a haematoma of 7 to 10 days.

198 CT scan of massive pontaneous intracerebral haemorrhage arising from the perforators on the left-side.

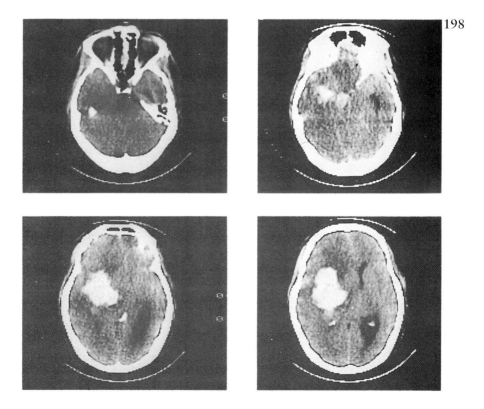

199

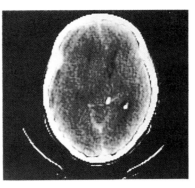

199 CT scan of a chronic left-sided subdural haematoma.

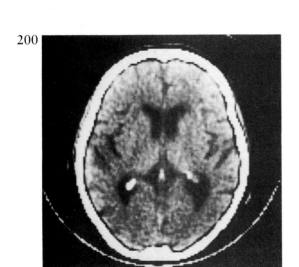

200 CT scan of a patient with dementia.
There is diffuse cerebral atrophy with widening of the fissures and some ventricular dilatation.

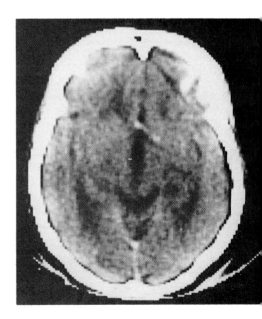

201 CT scan of multi-infarct dementia. There is well-marked hydrocephalus with multifocal areas of reduced attenuation in the periventricular white matter. The third ventricle is slightly enlarged. The fourth ventricle does not appear to be displaced. These features indicate atrophy secondary to multifocal ischaemic areas.

Angiography

Aortic arch angiography is an established procedure for visualising the great vessels in the neck. It will show atheroma, stenosis and thrombosis, and has a morbidity of 1%. Angiography should be carried out only if a specific type of treatment depends on its results. It is essential before surgery, e.g. carotid endarterectomy.

Angiography is contraindicated in patients with severe heart disease, chronic bronchitis, uncontrolled hypertension and in elderly patients who may have other disabilities.

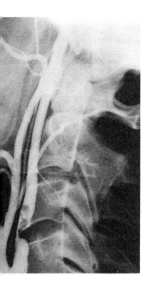
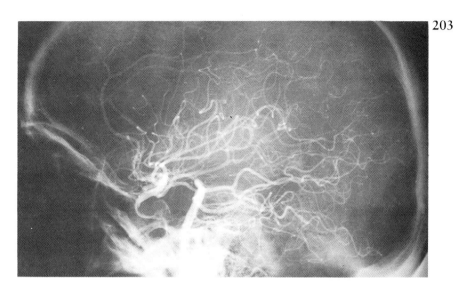

203

202 Angiogram showing stenosis of the internal carotid artery with thrombus and ulceration.

203 Angiogram of left internal carotid artery occlusion. There is collateral circulation via the posterior communicating artery.

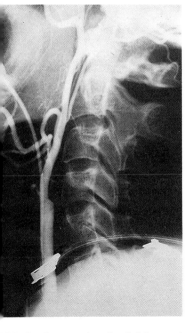
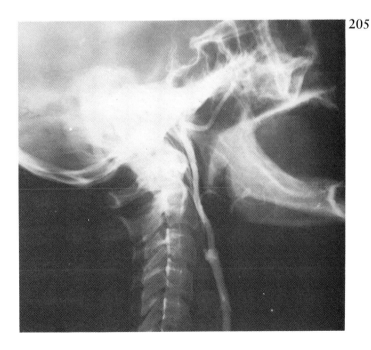

205

204 Angiogram showing left internal carotid artery occlusion.

205 Unsubtracted film showing internal carotid occlusion.

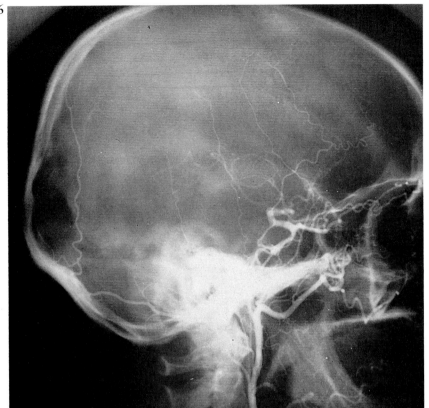

206 Unsubtracted film showing anastomotic circulation in a case of internal carotid artery occlusion.

207 Subtracted film showing external to internal carotid anastomosis secondary to internal carotid artery occlusion.

208 Angiogram showing a spondylitic spur displacing the vertebral artery. The patient may have symptoms of vertebrobasilar ischaemia.

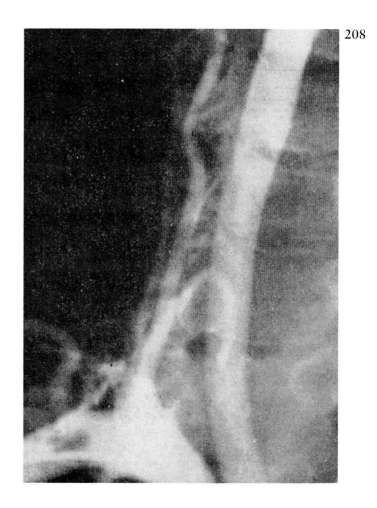

208

209 a) Chest tomogram showing a pulmonary arteriovenous malformation.

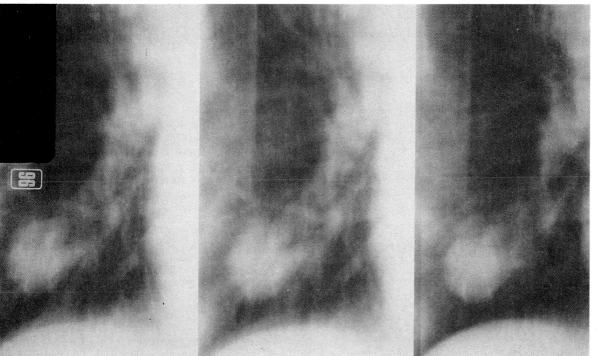

209a

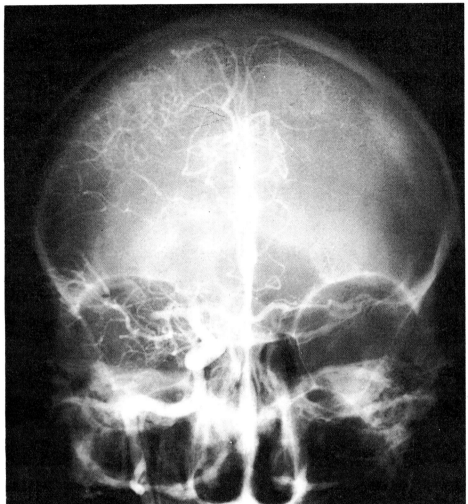

209 b) **Angiogram in same patient as shown in 209a,** showing left middle cerebral artery occlusion caused by embolus secondary to arteriovenous malformation.

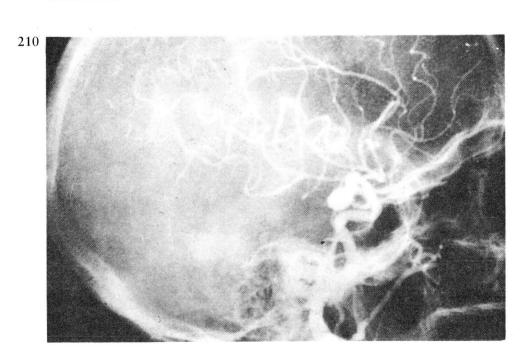

210 **Right carotid arteriogram showing a supraclinoid aneurysm** of the internal carotid artery at the origin of the posterior communicating artery.

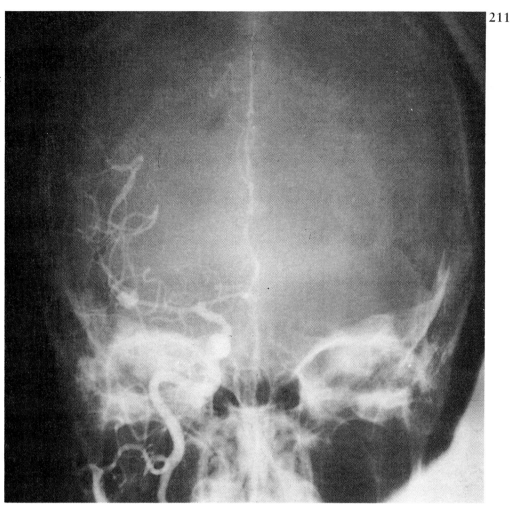

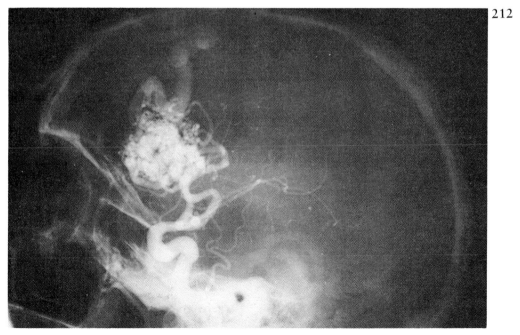

211 Angiogram showing middle cerebral artery aneurysm associated with haemorrhage and marked spasm of the middle and anterior cerebral arteries.

212 Arteriovenous malformation fed by an enlarged middle cerebral artery.

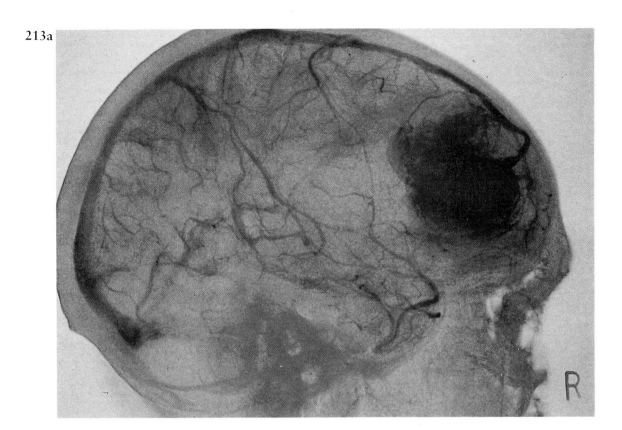

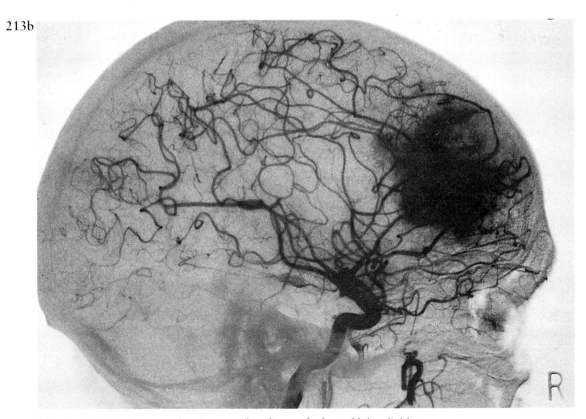

213 a) and b) Angiograms showing vascular phases of a frontal lobe glioblastoma.

214 Angiogram showing tumour vascularity of a large meningioma supplied by hypertrophied middle meningeal artery.

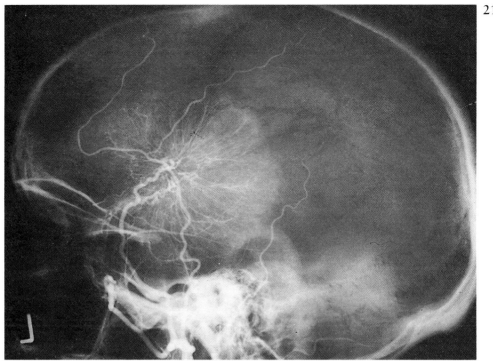

215 Angiogram showing a meningioma with a hypertrophied middle meningeal artery and the vascular tumour blush.

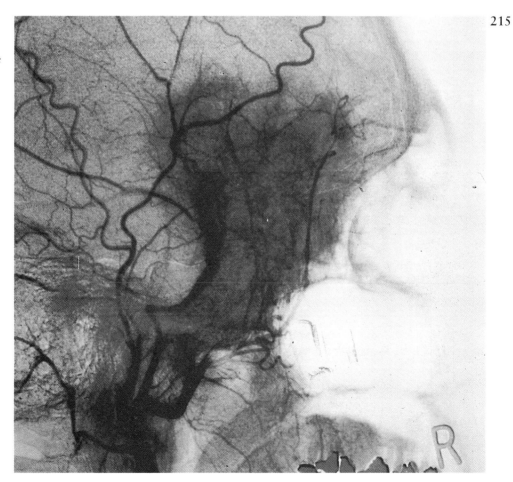

Non-invasive investigations

These techniques are in the early stages of development and are not widely available. Their value in the practical management of stroke has not been fully established.

1. Doppler continuous wave imaging

This involves continuous scanning of the course of extracranial arteries from the supraclavicular to the submandibular region. The instrument produces an image on the screen showing a flow map of the vessel. With this technique it is possible to detect size, extent and location of arterial lesions.

2. Oculoplethysmography

This technique depends upon recording the arterial pulse wave reaching each eyeball and measuring the small changes in the volume of the globe. Pulse arrival times at each eye can be compared. Delays of more than 40% above normal may occur with internal carotid stenosis.

3. Carotid phonangiography

A sensitive microphone is used to detect bruits over the carotids. These are then analysed for amplitude and frequency. Stenosis of less than 40% is not reliably detected.

4. Supraorbital Doppler recording

In this method a directional recorder is used to assess the velocity and direction of blood flow in the supraorbital artery. The ophthalmic artery (which is a branch of the internal carotid) communicates with the superficial temporal artery via the supraorbital artery. The superficial temporal artery is a branch of the external carotid artery and normally the blood flow is from the ophthalmic artery outwards to the superficial temporal artery. In cases of internal carotid artery stenosis the blood flow is reversed.

5. Pulsed Doppler imaging

This is a sophisticated technique and requires expensive equipment such as the MAVIS–C blood flow computer. Flow maps of the carotid and vertebral arteries may be imaged and atheroma can be localised.

6. Duplex scanning

This technique is a combination of real-time B-mode imaging and a pulsed Doppler ultrasound meter. The images are produced by the transducer scan and show moving arterial wall and measure of blood flow. The size and consistency of atheroma may be assessed and occlusion or stenosis of the lumen of greater than 50% can be diagnosed.

Digital subtraction angiography

In this procedure, carotid vessels are visualised to the same extent as with arteriography but the risks are minimised by using an intravenous route for injecting contrast medium. With an image intensifier and fast digital signal processing, pictures of very high quality are obtained. The use of the venous route avoids the risk of embolisation. It can be carried out in patients with severe atheroma and also those in whom conventional arteriography is contraindicated.

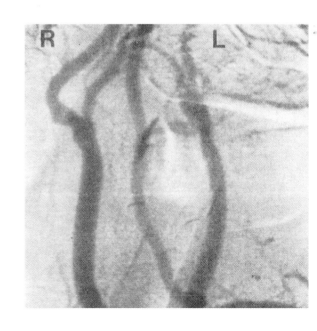

216 Digital subtraction angiogram showing irregular atheromatous plaque of the right internal carotid artery.

217 Digital subtraction angiogram showing stenosing **atheroma** of proximal left internal carotid artery, possibly with a large ulcer.

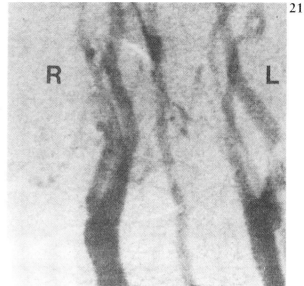

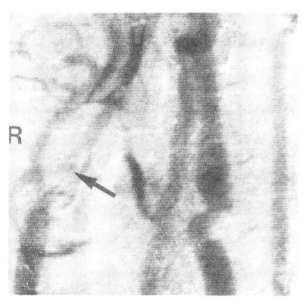

218 Digital subtraction angiogram showing stenosing **atheroma** at the bifurcation of the left common carotid and proximal internal carotid arteries; the external carotid artery is almost completely superimposed in this view. However, there is a severe stenosis of the right internal carotid artery (arrowed), although this is not so well visualised because of movements having occurred in the overlying larynx.

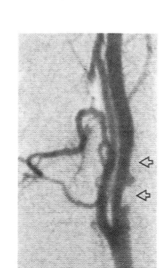

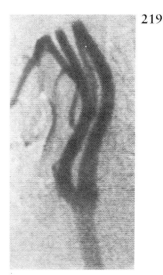

219

219 Digital subtraction angiogram study demonstrating irregular proximal internal carotid lesion (left) and normal contralateral vessel (right).

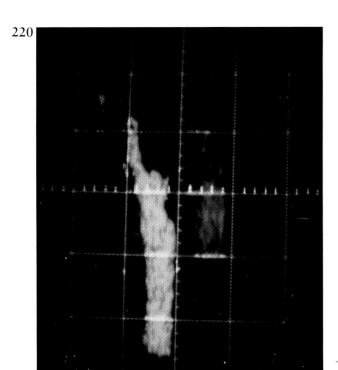 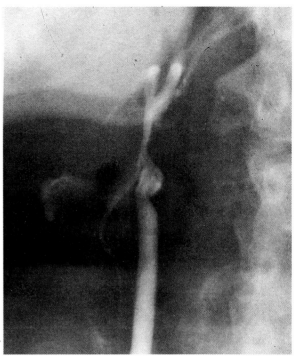

220 A MAVIS–C carotid image showing carotid stenosis with corresponding arteriogram.

TREATMENT OF STROKE

Most patients with acute stroke are initially treated in hospital.

The aims of treatment are to:

- Preserve the neurones surrounding the ischaemic brain tissue.
- Reduce the associated cerebral oedema.
- Maintain cerebral blood flow.
- Treat hypoxia and avoid hypercapnia.
- Treat seizures.
- Initiate early rehabilitation.
- Prevent complications.

Medical assessment

This starts with taking a full history and making an accurate diagnosis. A thorough medical assessment may require several sessions with the patient and/or relatives.

In the past history, check for diabetes, hypertension, heart disease, head injury, epilepsy, dementia, faints, TIAs and claudication.

The social background is important as it will have a bearing on rehabilitation. Check for marital status, type of housing, steps and stairs, whether living alone, any relatives, and any social support. In elderly patients, further details should be obtained from relatives, neighbours, health visitor and district nurse.

Medical examination

Medical examination is conducted along standard lines. Particular attention should be paid to the central nervous system. Detailed assessment is made of level of consciousness, hemiplegia, hemianaesthesia, hemianopia, speech defects and mental state. Also check for hypertension or hypotension, take the blood pressure in both arms to exclude 'subclavian steal', check for swallowing defects, breathing pattern, congestive heart failure, dysrhythmias, neck bruits (13% of patients over the age of 45 years have neck bruits), cardiac murmurs, peripheral vascular disease, temporal arteritis, anaemia, polycythaemia, hydration, breast masses, hepatomegaly and disturbed vision. Also examine the fundi (for hypertensive retinopathy, papilloedema, subhyaloid haemorrhage),

and do a rectal examination to exclude faecal impaction.

Differential diagnosis of neck bruits includes carotid stenosis, venous hums, aortic stenosis and mitral incompetence.

Assessment of consciousness level (after Teasdale and Jennett[4])

The level of consciousness should be assessed immediately after admission and then at regular intervals. For accuracy, a standard procedure should be followed, such as the one shown here:

- Pulse.
- Blood pressure.
- Respiration — rate, type.
- Temperature — ?rectal.
- Pupils — size, equality, reaction.
- Eye opening:
  Spontaneous
  To speech
  To pain
  None
- Best verbal response:
  Orientated
  Confused
  Inappropriate
  Incomprehensible
  None
- Best motor response (right and left):
  Obeying
  Localising
  Flexing
  Extending
  None

Assessment of neurological deficit

Typical hemiplegic posture consists of:

- Head and gaze towards the side of the lesion.
- Leg in extension.
- Foot in plantar flexion.
- Arm pronated and flexed across the chest.
- Fingers flexed.

Other CNS features vary according to the type and extent of the cerebral lesion:

- Pupillary abnormalities.
- Abnormalities of eye movements.
- Horner's syndrome.
- Loss of corneal reflex.
- Homonymous hemianopia.
- Loss of gag reflex.
- Abnormalities of deglutition.
- Facial palsy.
- Dysphasia and dysarthria.
- Sensory changes — these can contribute to the development of pressure sores and shoulder dislocation.
- Perceptual problems — usually with lesions of the right non-dominant hemisphere. Neglect of left half of space.

Functional assessment

Functional assessment should be made in stroke survivors before and then at regular intervals throughout the period of rehabilitation.

The following points are noted:

Mental state. Orientation, memory, comprehension, ability to read and write, perseveration, behaviour, motivation, emotions, confidence, insight, body perception and dementia.

General health. Ischaemic heart disease, congestive heart failure, chronic airways disease, osteoarthritis, peripheral vascular disease, and musculoskeletal disorders.

Autonomic function. Incontinence, constipation, urinary tract infection, postural hypotension, shoulder–hand syndrome.

Special senses. Vision, hearing, speech, cataracts, use of spectacles or hearing aid, dysphasia, dysarthria, swallowing difficulties, state of dentures.

Posture control. Check for the patient's ability to maintain balance while sitting, standing and walking.

Motor deficits. Severity and extent of paralysis. Also check for spasticity, clonus, exaggerated reflexes and hemiplegic gait.

Sensory deficits. Check sensory system, postural sensation and disorders of body image, spatial sensation, apraxia and agnosia.

Medical management

Acute stroke is a medical emergency. Investigations should be arranged as soon as possible. Medical and nursing management begins immediately after admission to hospital.

An **unconscious patient** should be nursed lying on his side, and there should be easy access to resuscitative equipment. Ensure that the airway is free and that there are no secretions at the back of the throat. Also check for loose dentures and displaced tongue. Bulbar palsy and irregular breathing indicate a poor prognosis.

Ensure **adequate hydration** with good urinary output (catheterise if necessary). Nursing care should include frequent turning and care of the mouth and eyes.

Consider **antibiotics** for chest infection, but in very elderly patients there may be ethical objections. If a patient has had a major stroke with severe neurological deficit then there must be doubts about using active resuscitive measures.

Poor prognosis is indicated by:

- Unconsciousness.
- Old age.
- Hypertension.
- Confusion or dementia.
- Unequal pupils.
- Cheyne–Stokes breathing.
- Bilateral CNS signs.
- Second or third stroke.
- Chest infection.

Cerebral blood flow can be increased, but this may result in blood being directed away from the area that is already ischaemic. In cases with hypotension, one should gently raise the blood pressure, as cerebral blood flow to ischaemic areas might be improved. If there is extreme hypertension then a slow reduction of systolic blood pressure to about 180 mm Hg is advisable (by means of intravenous mannitol or careful use of antihypertensive drugs).

Hypoxia carries a high mortality. This can be treated by improving oxygenation — clearing the airways, giving oxygen (sometimes hyperbaric oxygen) and chest physiotherapy.

Medical management during the acute phase will include treatment of other associated diseases such as diabetes and chronic bronchitis, and careful monitoring of blood pressure, respiration, urea, electrolytes and blood gases.

Acute cerebral infarction

General measures are the same as those for any unconscious patient, i.e. bed rest, careful positioning, intravenous fluids, suction, maintenance of airway, and antibiotics. Combined medical and nursing skills are required. In middle-aged and young patients, aim to maintain the diastolic blood pressure between 90 and 100 mm Hg, with appropriate drugs, e.g. hydralazine, diazoxide.

Cerebral vasodilators. The role of these drugs remains unclear and it is doubtful whether they have any use in acute stroke. Naftidrofuryl and isoxsuprine have been tried but results are conflicting.

Cerebral oedema. This extends the neurological damage and attempts should be made to reduce it. Dexamethasone (beginning with 4 mg 6-hourly), intravenous mannitol, frusemide, glycerol and Dextran 40 have all been used, but the exact benefits are still not clear. The possibility that calcium entry blocking agents might help in ischaemic brain damage is being extensively investigated.

Subarachnoid haemorrhage

Diagnosis is confirmed by a lumbar puncture. CT scan and angiographic studies are done, especially if surgery is being considered. Restlessness and agitation are common and mild sedation may be required. Conscious patients may complain of severe headache, which will need a strong analgesic. Surgery may consist of clipping an aneurysm and evacuation of surrounding haematoma. In some patients ligation of the internal carotid artery may reduce the risk of bleeding from an aneurysm. Small angiomatous malformations may be amenable to surgery.

Intracerebral haemorrhage

Patients are usually very ill and the prognosis is poor. A CT scan will confirm the diagnosis. Attempts should be made to reduce cerebral oedema with dexamethasone or diuretics. Rarely, an intracerebral haematoma may be removed surgically, but the prognosis remains poor.

Cerebral embolism

Patients with cerebral infarction caused by embolism usually have an underlying disorder such as mitral stenosis with atrial fibrillation, recent myocardial infarction, or bacterial endocarditis. In selected patients, long-term anticoagulant therapy will reduce the risk of subsequent cerebral embolism. Anticoagulants are contraindicated in bacterial endocarditis and in patients with haemorrhagic disorders. Occasionally, anticoagulant therapy may cause a haemorrhage into a recent infarct. Anticoagulants may be useful in certain selected patients with TIAs.

Management of TIAs

(See also 'clinical manifestations', page 40, and chapter on investigations, page 70.) Make an accurate diagnosis and exclude focal epilepsy, drop attacks, hysteria, syncope, etc. Identify associated risk factors, such as anaemia, diabetes, hypertension, cardiac dysrhythmia and valvular heart disease. In 25% of patients, no obvious cause is found.

Investigations include:

- Haemoglobin, full blood count and ESR.

- Platelet count.

- Blood sugar estimation.

- Standard ECG and a 24-hour ECG (to exclude transient cardiac arrhythmias).

- Echocardiography may show valvular deformity.

- EEG may be required to exclude cases of focal epilepsy.

- X-ray of the chest may show evidence of cardiac or pulmonary disease.

- X-ray of the skull is usually done for medicolegal reasons when a patient has fallen (with TIA) and sustained a head injury. Calcification of the carotid siphon may be seen.

- Isotope scan may show cerebral infarction, cerebral tumours or subdural haematoma.

- CT scan should ideally be done in every case of TIA. Primary gliomas, meningiomas and cerebral metastases can all present with transient neurological episodes. Small infarcts, angiomas and aneurysms may be seen.

- Angiography. This is the recognised procedure for assessing disease of blood vessels in the neck and cerebral circulation. It is essential before contemplating surgery.

Treatment of TIAs

General measures, such as treatment of anaemia, cardiac failure, polycythaemia, hypertension, mitral stenosis.

Drugs. *Anticoagulants:* the usefulness of anticoagulants in preventing TIAs or a major stroke remains doubtful. However, in selected patients there may be some benefit in giving anticoagulants for a period of 6 months after a TIA. If there is a known source of emboli, such as mitral stenosis with atrial fibrillation, then anticoagulants must be given. TIAs caused by emboli from carotid atheroma also benefit from long-term anticoagulation.

Antiplatelet drugs: trials have shown that aspirin in small doses given to men, especially those under 55 years of age, is effective in reducing platelet adhesion and thus preventing TIAs. Dipyridamole may also have some benefit and has been found to be effective in reducing emboli from prosthetic cardiac valves. Oxpentifylline, which improves peripheral circulation, has been tried in cerebral vascular disorders, with promising results.

If there is an obvious source of emboli in a young or middle-aged patient, then anticoagulants should be considered. If the source of emboli is unknown or if there are contraindications to anticoagulants, then antiplatelet drugs may be used.

Surgery. In carefully selected patients surgery is effective in treating TIAs. Stenotic lesions of the internal carotid artery are treated by endarterectomy. If stenosis is extensive and long then a permanent bypass graft may be considered. A blocked artery can be bypassed by a shunt.

If there is involvement of the carotid siphon and of the middle cerebral artery and this is giving rise to TIAs, then an extracranial–intracranial anastomosis may be considered. The anastomosis is performed between a branch of the superficial temporal artery and a branch of the middle cerebral artery. The aim of the operation is to bypass the occlusion in the internal carotid artery and thus improve blood flow to the cerebral hemisphere. Further experience is required before the exact value of this operation becomes clear in the treatment and prevention of TIAs and strokes.

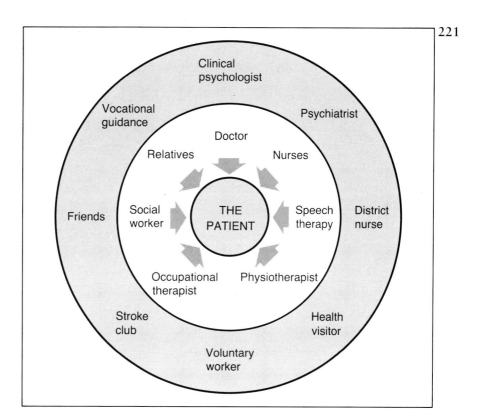

221 A multidisciplinary approach is an essential ingredient of successful stroke rehabilitation.

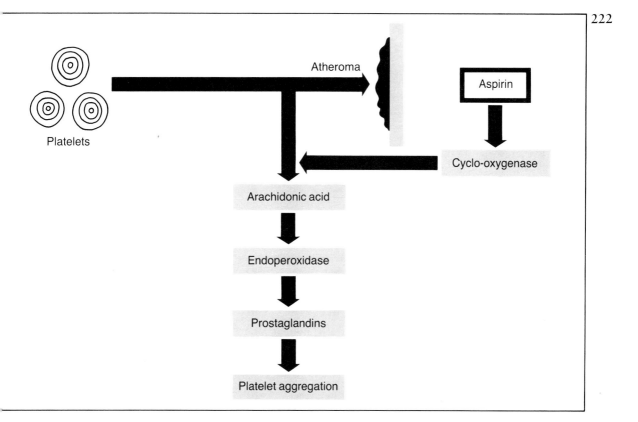

222 Aspirin and dipyridamole reduce platelet stickiness and are useful in treating TIAs. Aspirin blocks the enzymatic steps that lead to increased platelet aggregation.

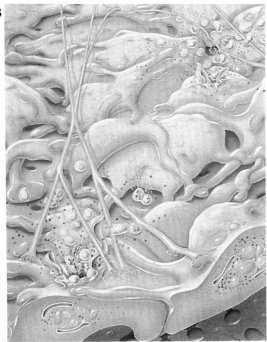

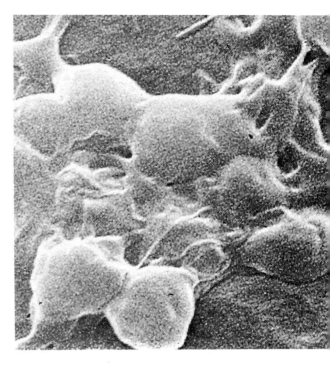

223 Three-dimensional representation of irreversible platelet aggregation initiated by the release of serotonin and adenosine diphosphate (ADP).

224 Scanning electron microscope picture showing platelet aggregation. Oxpentifylline has also been shown to reduce platelet aggregation.

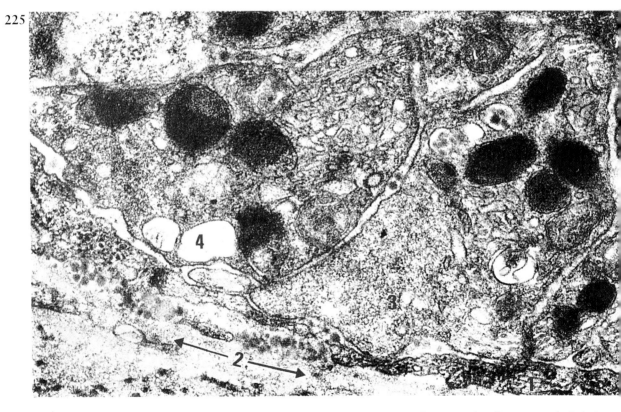

225 This electron micrograph shows an enlarged detail of platelets aggregated at a vessel wall (1). An endothelial lesion (2) covered by two platelets (3 and 4) is clearly visible in the centre of the picture.

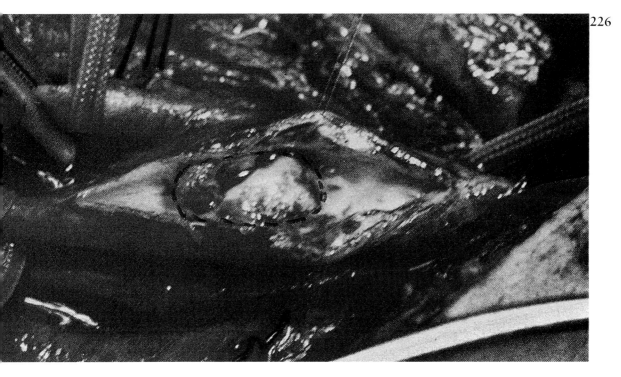

226 Opened internal carotid artery showing ball thrombus occluding the lumen (endarterectomy).

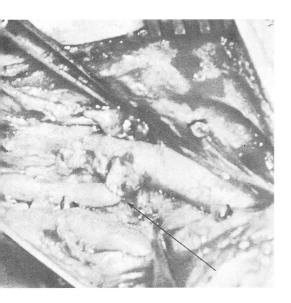

227 Operative photograph of reconstructed internal carotid artery using autogenous saphenous vein. The proximal suture line is clearly visible.

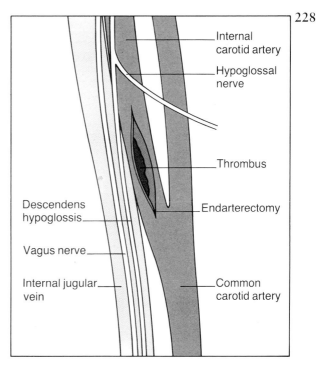

228 Carotid endarterectomy. Important structures in relation to the internal carotid artery are shown, along with a thrombus in its lumen.

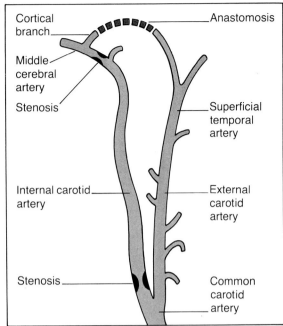

229 **Intracranial to extracranial anastomosis** — between a cortical branch of the middle cerebral artery and a branch of the superficial temporal artery.

Patient management after the acute phase

(See also chapter on rehabilitation, page 147.)

After the acute phase the management becomes less intensive, but it is important that the physician in charge takes a continuing interest in the patient and acts as the leader of the rehabilitation team. Following the acute stage of illness, the patient should be mobilised. He should participate in the ward activities and should not be placed in an isolated position.

Active rehabilitation begins with a multi-disciplinary team approach. Attention should be paid to other coexisting disabilities (particularly in an elderly patient), e.g. arthritis, deafness, dementia, parkinsonism, bronchitis, peripheral vascular disease and cardiac failure. Before initiating a programme of long-term rehabilitation, the patient should be assessed by the following people:

- Occupational therapist.
- Physiotherapist.
- Social worker.
- Speech therapist.
- Clinical psychologist (if available).

It is important that the patient is not burdened by too many complexities during rehabilitation, or by too many people, as this will be intimidating and counterproductive.

Attention should be directed at preventing and treating complications. If the patient is on an acute ward, then further rehabilitation may be arranged in a different department. For this the patient may have to be transferred to a geriatric rehabilitation ward, stroke unit, young chronic disabled unit or neurological rehabilitation department. Many patients will be able to go home and continue with their further therapy as an outpatient. If the patient's stay at home is to be successful, the domiciliary physiotherapist, district nurse, social worker, general practitioner, the patient's family and day hospitals will be of crucial importance. Further details are given in the chapter on rehabilitation.

Complications following a stroke

Complications include:

- Pressure sores.
- Respiratory tract infections.
- Urinary incontinence.
- Constipation.
- Deep vein thrombosis.
- Spasticity and contractures.
- Pain in the shoulder (frozen shoulder).
- Psychiatric problems.
- Miscellaneous.

Pressure sores

Superficial — good prognosis if treated actively. Deep — tissue necrosis. Prognosis poor.

Compression and shearing forces initiate the tissue injury.

Predisposing factors

- Poor tissue perfusion.
- Immobility and paresis.
- Hypoxaemia.
- Urinary and faecal incontinence.
- Abrasive bed sheets.
- Poor general health — congestive cardiac failure, hypotension, anaemia.

Management of pressure sores

- Skin care — regular turning with lifting. Avoid shearing. Inspect pressure areas regularly.

Table 1 Exton-Smith's clinical score for patients at risk of pressure sores.[5] (Patients scoring over 7 points are at greater risk.)

General condition	Mental state	Activity	Mobility	Incontinence
0 – Good	0 – Alert	0 – Ambulant	0 – Full	0 – None
1 – Fair	1 – Confused	1 – Walks	1 – Slightly impaired	1 – Occasional
2 – Poor	2 – Apathetic	2 – Chairfast	2 – Greatly impaired	2 – Incontinent of urine
3 – Bad	3 – Stuporous	3 – Bedfast	3 – Immobile	3 – Doubly incontinent

Judicious use of sheepskin pads and boots, ripple beds, absorbent sheets, net suspension bed, flotation mattresses, etc.

- Catheterise if patient is persistently incontinent.

- Use bed cradles.

- Wash the skin gently with soap and water. Avoid rubbing.

Superficial sores. Avoid further pressure and contact with faeces and urine. Use a light plastic dressing. One- or two-hourly turning. Treat associated conditions, such as anaemia, oedema, dehydration.

Deep sores. The patient's general health will need attention. Regular packing of pressure sore cavity with Eusol (1:2000) and paraffin is helpful. Various products are available that will deslough and promote healing of the sore. Surgical debridement of necrotic tissue may be required. Sometimes oral metronidazole is used to clear anaerobic infection but this needs to be given for a prolonged period. In selected patients plastic surgery should be considered.

Respiratory tract infections

Aspiration and hypostatic pneumonia occur, especially in patients with swallowing difficulties. Prevention is by early mobilisation, breathing exercises and chest physiotherapy. Broad-spectrum antibiotics will be required for treatment.

Urinary incontinence (See also chapter on nursing care, page 122)

Stroke patients become incontinent for various reasons. Neurological disorders cause different types of urinary incontinence. Elderly stroke patients tend to develop incontinence as a result of neurogenic bladder caused by a lesion of the higher centres in the frontal lobe. In some patients there may be other contributory factors, such as diabetic neuropathy, dementia, cystitis, senile vaginitis and prostatic hypertrophy.

Management of urinary incontinence
First find the cause. Carry out a rectal and a vaginal examination and check urine for sugar and infection.

The frequency and pattern of incontinence should be noted on a 24-hour chart. Frequent toileting in privacy and the use of bedside commodes with habit training will control many cases of incontinence.

In men, persistent incontinence and dribbling can be managed by a system of condom drainage. Sporran and sheath-type urinals are useful in long-term care. Female patients can be kept dry with marsupial pants or stretch pants with pads.

In some patients permanent catheterisation will be the only solution. Elderly patients with indwelling catheters are prone to frequent urinary tract infections. Such patients should be given antibiotics only if there are systemic symptoms and/or signs of renal involvement.

Frequent bladder washouts will reduce the incidence of infections and also prevent recurrent catheter blockage.

Constipation

Untreated constipation leads to faecal impaction and overflow faecal incontinence. The diagnosis is made by rectal examination and plain x-ray of the abdomen.

Management consists of early activity, adequate hydration, high-fibre diet and laxatives. Severe constipation will require suppositories, enemata or manual removal of faeces.

Deep vein thrombosis (DVT)

Over 50% of stroke patients suffer a DVT in the paralysed leg. Low-dose heparin and elastic graduated pressure stockings are useful aids in prevention. A massive DVT should be treated with bed rest, analgesia and anticoagulants.

The diagnosis of pulmonary embolism is confirmed by plain x-ray of the chest and/or an isotope lung scan.

Spasticity and contractures

These are usually caused by defective posture, poor positioning and inadequate rehabilitation. Prolonged physiotherapy may ease the spasticity but contractures are more difficult to treat. Commonly used drugs are baclofen, dantrolene and diazepam. In cases where there is severe pain and deformity, surgery may be considered.

Pain in the shoulder (frozen shoulder)

Pain and stiffness in the shoulder of a hemiplegic patient may result from several different causes:

- Impacted fracture of the neck of the humerus sustained during the fall at the time of stroke.
- Rotator cuff injury.
- Diastasis of the shoulder joint because of the weight of the arm during the flaccid stage of hemiplegia.
- Contracture.
- Post-hemiplegic reflex sympathetic dystrophy.
- Heterotopic calcification of the shoulder joint.
- Supraspinatus tendinitis.
- Adhesive capsulitis.
- Brachial plexus injury.

The management of painful shoulder depends on the underlying cause. Accurate diagnosis is important. In many hemiplegics frozen shoulder can be prevented with early physiotherapy, correct positioning of the paralysed arm and correct handling of the patient. Later, the treatment includes stretching exercises, serial splinting, intra-articular injections and heat therapy.

Psychiatric problems

These are more frequent in male patients with multi-infarct dementia and those with right hemisphere lesions. Confusion, restlessness and emotional lability are common. Some patients develop severe depression, bereavement-like reactions, apathy, paranoid psychosis, aggressiveness and antisocial habits.

Multidisciplinary management is necessary and will include careful use of sedatives, tranquillizers and hypnotics. Nursing care and occupational therapy are of vital importance. Relatives and a clinical psychologist can give useful help in management. Severely disturbed patients will require psychiatric assessment.

Miscellaneous complications

- Oedema of the paralysed limb.
- Reversal of sleeping habits.
- Malnutrition secondary to pseudobulbar palsy.
- Postural hypotension.
- Long thoracic nerve palsy — wing scapula.
- Ulnar nerve palsy — drop wrist.
- Median nerve palsy.
- Reflex dystrophy of the hand.
- Foot drop.
- Sciatic neuropathy — caused by prolonged pressure over the sciatic notch in an immobile patient.
- Hyperextension of the knee.
- Perceptual problems.
- Epilepsy in up to 15% of patients.
- Osteoporosis in the paralysed limb.
- Torticollis.
- Complete loss of posture and balance.
- Fractured neck of femur, especially in the elderly, because of frequent falls.

230 Large pressure sore in an elderly patient with dense right hemiplegia.

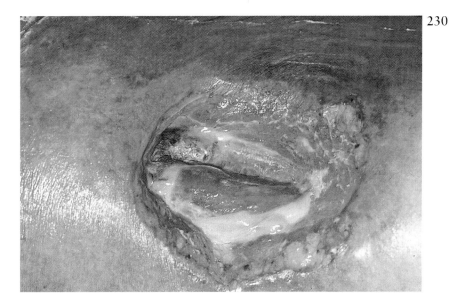

231 Pressure sore on the heel – a frequent problem with immobile stroke patients who may also have peripheral vascular disease.

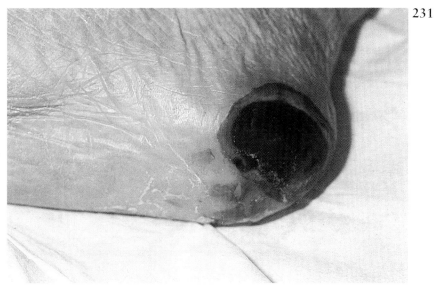

232 Skin rash caused by urinary incontinence.

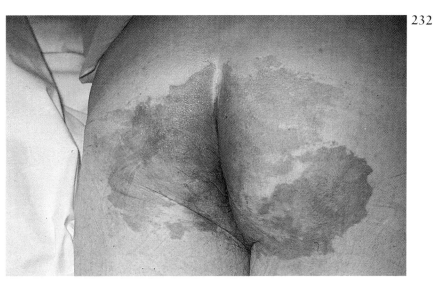

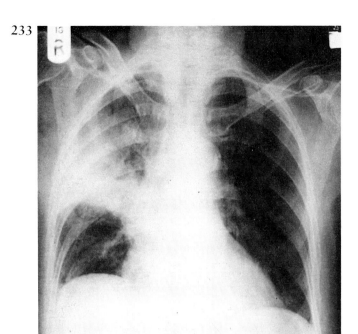

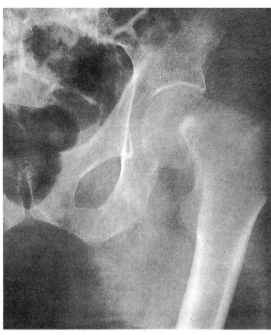

233 **Right-sided chest infection** in a patient with pseudobulbar palsy.

234 **Fractured neck of left femur** sustained when the patient fell during a transient ischaemic attack.

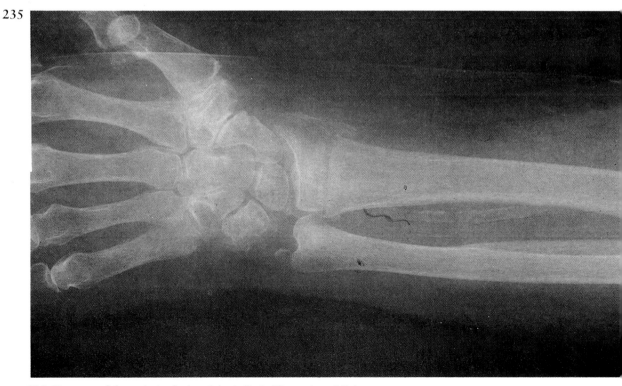

235 **Fracture of the wrist** in the hemiplegic limb. The patient fell during attempts at walking.

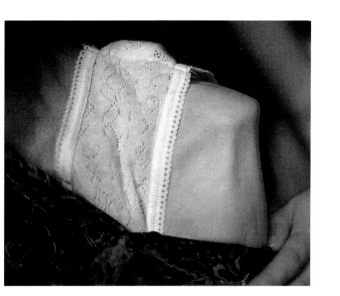

236 Subluxation of the glenohumeral joint of the hemiplegic left arm.

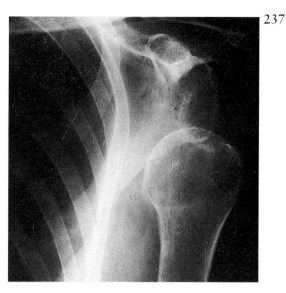

237 X-ray showing subluxation of the glenohumeral joint.

238 Impacted fracture of the neck of the humerus giving rise to shoulder pain in a patient with left hemiplegia.

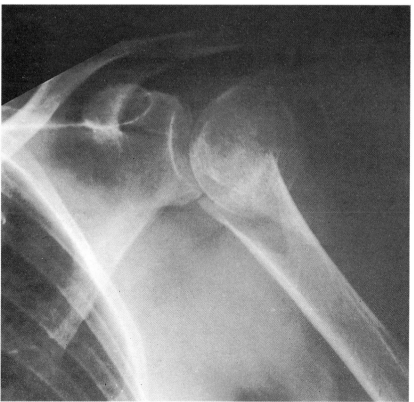

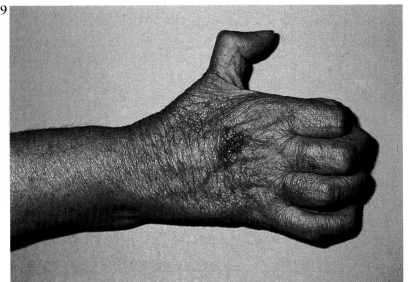

239 Claw-hand deformity caused by ulnar nerve palsy.

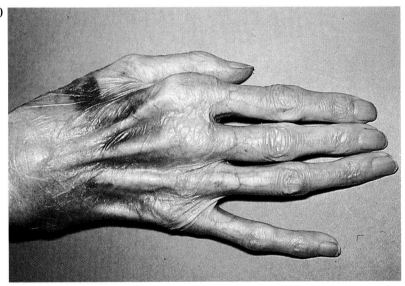

240 Wasting of the small muscles of the hand in a patient with long-standing hemiplegia.

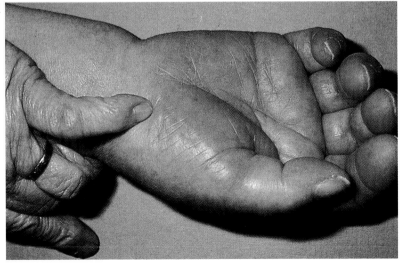

241 Autonomic changes in a hemiplegic hand, which is swollen, spastic and tender (reflex sympathetic dystrophy).

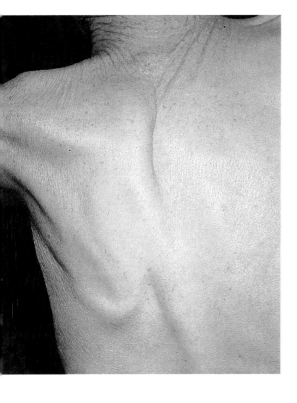

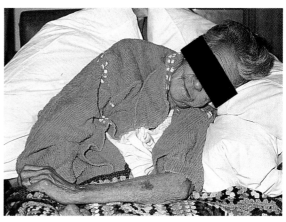

243 Complete loss of posture in a patient who has had several cerebrovascular episodes.

242 Wing scapula caused by long thoracic nerve palsy.
This can occur when the weak arm is allowed to hang over the side of the chair or between the rails of the cot-side.

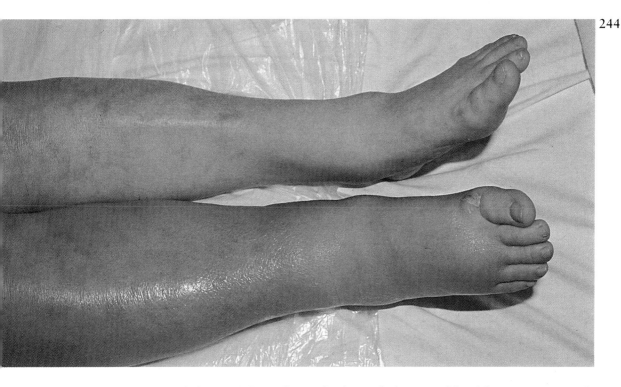

244 Deep vein thrombosis of the right leg. Note the swelling and redness. The leg is painful and the patient is pyrexial.

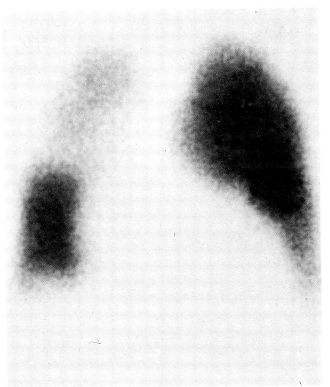

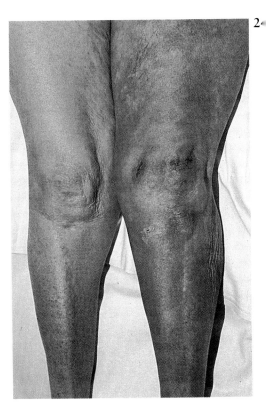

245 Ventilation perfusion pulmonary scan showing reduced perfusion to the upper half of the right lung. Appearances are of pulmonary embolism following a DVT.

246 Left femoral artery thrombosis in a patient with left hemiplegia and cardiac failure.

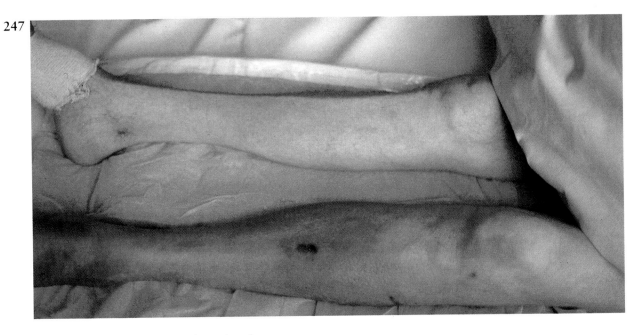

247 Cellulitis developing in the hemiplegic leg.

248 Frozen shoulder in a
patient with left hemiplegia.
It is caused by adhesive
capsulitis, which is a frequent
complication of a stroke.

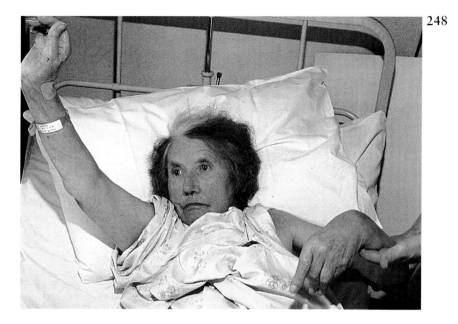

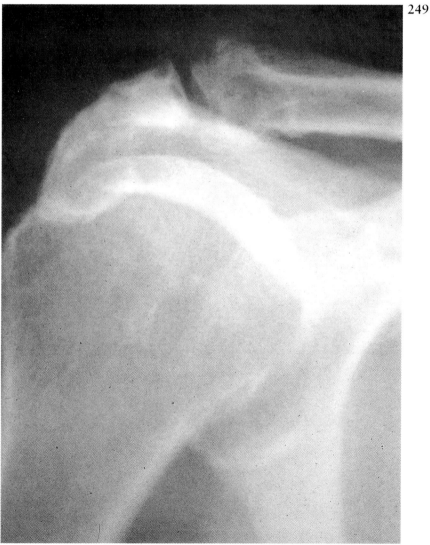

249 X-ray of frozen shoulder
caused by supraspinatus
tendinitis. Note the calcification
in the supraspinatus tendon.

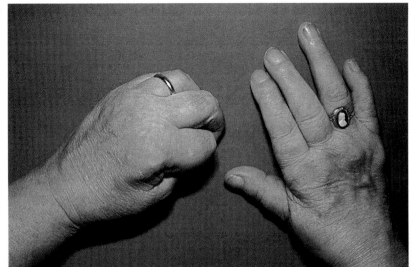

250 Severe **contracture** of the left hand several months after a dense hemiplegia.

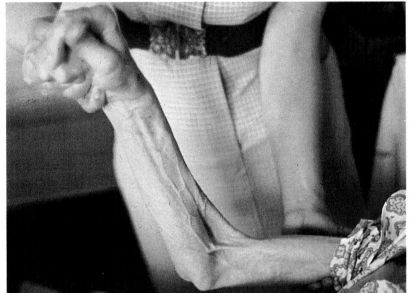

251 Spasticity in a hemiplegic arm.

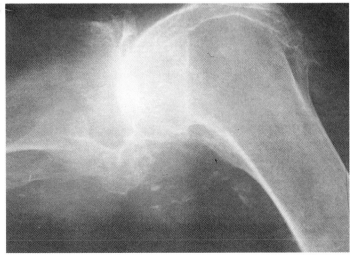

252 X-ray of the knee showing flexion contracture, osteoarthritis and heterotopic calcification in the hemiplegic leg.

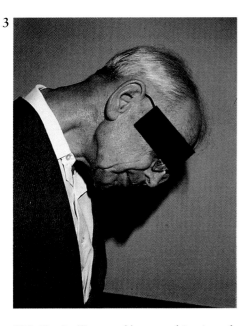

253 Torticollis caused by a combination of severe stroke, lack of motivation, dementia, poor posture control and inadequate rehabilitation.

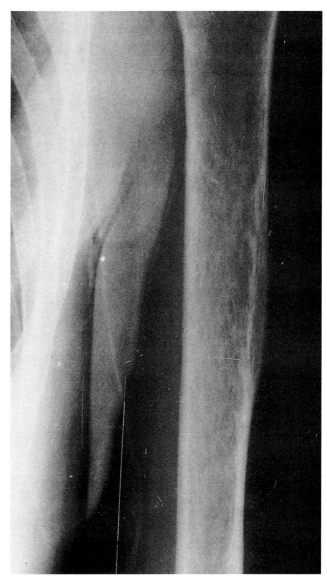

254 Osteoporosis in a hemiplegic humerus — there is risk of stress fracture. ▶

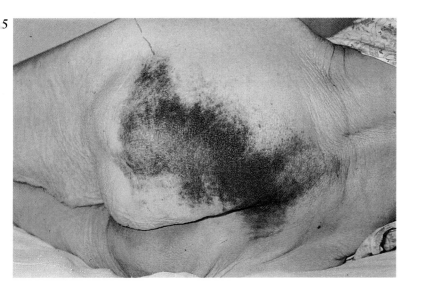

255 Severe bruising over the sacrum and left buttock sustained at the time of stroke when the patient fell.

256

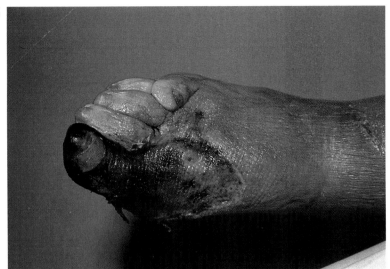

256 Ischaemic necrosis caused by severe peripheral vascular disease. The patient had also suffered from a cerebral infarction.

257

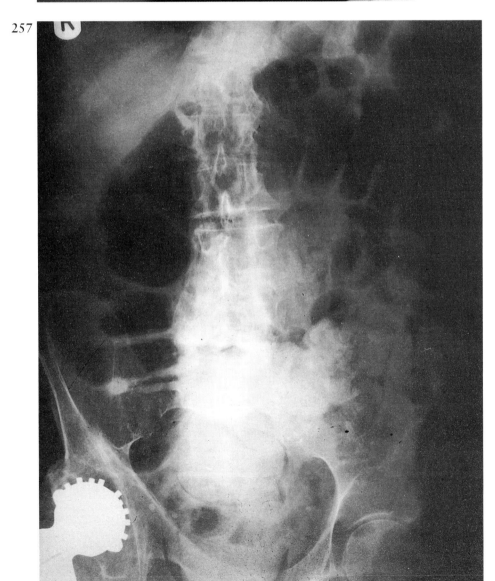

257 Intestinal obstruction caused by faecal impaction in a patient immobile with a right hemiplegia.

258 **Poor oral hygiene** resulting candidiasis in a stroke patient.

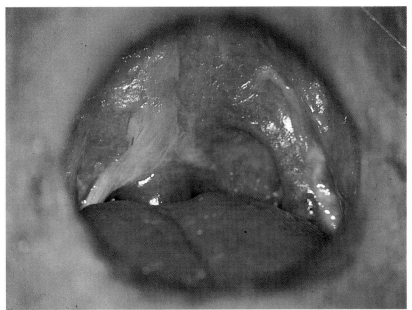

Prognosis after stroke

Cerebral infarction accounts for about 80% of stroke cases. Mortality within the first month of cerebral infarction is between 25 and 40%.

Haemorrhage occurs in 20%.

Level of consciousness is the most important sign in predicting the immediate outcome after stroke. In patients who remain fully conscious over the first 48 hours, the average mortality is less than 25%. Drowsy patients — over 50% die. Unconscious patients — about 75% die.

Recovery is usually poor in patients who have conjugate gaze paralysis and/or total flaccid hemiplegia.

50% of patients die within the first year after a stroke and 20 to 30% are permanently disabled.

Speech 'improves' in about 60% of patients, but full recovery may take up to 2 years.

The long-term outlook depends on several factors:
1 The site, size and nature of the lesion.
2 Age and sex.
3 General health.
4 Pre-morbid intelligence and personality.
5 Social circumstances.
6 Quality and quantity of available rehabilitation.

● Prognosis is poor with:
1 Old age.
2 Prolonged unconsciousness.
3 Persistent hypertension.
4 Confusion, dementia or depression.
5 Unequal pupils.
6 Irregular breathing patterns.
7 Bilateral CNS signs.
8 Second or third stroke.
9 Bronchopneumonia.
10 Conjugate gaze paralysis.
11 Widespread atheroma.
12 Cardiac failure.

NURSING CARE

Gillian Snowley

The successful management and rehabilitation of the stroke patient must be a team activity. Whilst medical and paramedical services make an important contribution, the patient spends most of his time directly with the nurse. The nurse is also likely to be the first contact with the stroke patient, and thus will set the tone of the recovery process.

To plan nursing care effectively, the nurse must be able to identify accurately where there are problems of maintaining sufficient quantity and quality of self-care for health and well being. In order to assess the need, plan, implement and evaluate nursing care, many nurses use an 'activities of living' model of nursing as the basis for care delivery (e.g. Henderson 1966[6]). Such a model forms the framework of this chapter.

The nursing management of the stroke patient may be divided into three main phases:

1 Maintaining processes essential to life.

2 Preventing complications and further loss of function.

3 Restoring as much function as possible to rebuild a productive life.

Maintaining processes essential to life

Respiration and cardiovascular function

At the beginning, the patient may be unconscious or very drowsy, and should be placed in the recovery position to prevent the tongue from falling back and obstructing the airway. Dentures, if present, should be removed. Occasionally, an artificial airway or even endotracheal intubation may be used. In some cases oxygen may be administered via a facial mask. Where a patient is conscious but has lost mobility and control over body posture, the nurse may need to help him achieve the best-position for lung ventilation. This may include judicious use of backrests, pillows and foam wedges. The use of pharyngeal/endotracheal suction, or encouragement to cough up sputum may be necessary to clear the airway. The role of the nurse in maintaining adequate cardiovascular function is largely supportive, i.e. in the administration of drugs and the recording of observations for effectiveness of treatment. For example, if antihypertensives are prescribed, blood pressure monitoring will be necessary. In addition, the nurse will need to give advice to the patient and his family to prevent unnecessary anxiety.

Adequate nutrition and hydration

If unconsciousness is prolonged or if the swallowing reflex is impaired, adequate nutrition and hydration may have to be maintained artificially. A nasogastric tube may be left in situ. Gradual retraining of the patient in using a spoon or drinking cup to take fluids should become part of every meal-time. Occasionally, intravenous therapy will be necessary to restore fluid and electrolyte balance. Observation and care of the cannula site will be necessary.

Throughout the period of artificial feeding, oral hygiene should be carried out to maintain a moist and healthy mouth.

Maintaining body temperature

In some cases of stroke, the patient's body temperature may be altered, either as a result of the brain damage or if the person has been lying immobilised for several hours. Temperature recording on admission is vital. Hypothermia, when the body temperature is below 35°C, should be treated using aluminium blankets, if available. Hyperpyrexia, which occurs when the heat regulating centre is impaired, can be reduced by tepid-sponging, use of fans, etc.

Vital nursing observations during the acute phase

Blood pressure and pulse recordings taken frequently following admission may give an indication of the state of intracranial pressure. Rising blood pressure and falling pulse rate indicate an increase in intracranial pressure. Where the stroke has been caused by intracranial haemorrhage, blood pressure recordings to indicate the degree of hypertension may be crucial.

The respiration rate and temperature recordings give valuable indication of progress.

Neurological observations are important. Pupil reactions and the patient's response levels to voice or painful stimuli should be recorded. These observations may indicate the early progress of the stroke.

Preventing complications and further loss of function

Respiration and cardiovascular function

Prolonged immobility of the stroke patient may lead to consolidation of secretions in the lungs, and circulatory stasis with the threat of venous thrombosis. Skilled positioning and regular changes of position will help ventilate the lungs, and removal of secretions by expectoration or suction will help to prevent pneumonia.

Regular passive exercising of all limbs three or four times a day should begin immediately. This improves venous return and helps to prevent venous thrombosis. The nurse should observe the thighs and calves of the stroke patient for signs of enlargement and tenderness, which may indicate a deep vein thrombosis.

Elimination of body waste

Micturition may be severely disrupted in stroke, resulting in incontinence in the acute phase, and this may become a permanent problem. The management of initial incontinence is often an important factor in the eventual achievement of good bladder control. Apart from its physical management, a positive, sympathetic and patient nurse will encourage achievement of good bladder control in the future. Catheterisation in the early stages of stroke is not recommended, as this makes bladder retraining more difficult, and indwelling catheters interefere with mobility and provide a potential route of infection. The use of incontinence pads or pants, with scrupulous skin care and linen changing is preferable. Male patients may be fitted with an external urine sheath and drainage bag. Where catheterisation is considered essential, a closed drainage system must be used, to try to prevent infection.

Incontinence of faeces is not a major problem in the early stages of management of the stroke patient, but constipation may necessitate the use of laxatives or suppositories.

Protection of the skin

The immobile stroke patient, particularly if there is sensory loss, may develop pressure sores. It is essential that the nursing staff make initial and subsequent assessments of the degree of risk. The Exton-Smith Scoring System of assessment is effective if used accurately (see page 109). In addition, pressure-measuring instruments are now available to assess the degree of pressure to which bony prominences are subjected. Careful use of this gauge will allow the nurse to provide the best possible pressure-relieving surface on which to nurse the patient. Special mattresses, beds, sheepskin or foam pads, may be provided according to the individual needs of the patient.

At all times the patient must be carefully handled to prevent scratching and scraping of the skin. Changing position regularly may be necessary to prevent prolonged and damaging pressure on any one area of skin. Hand rubbing of the pressure area should never be practised, as this is known to cause tissue damage.

Movement and maintenance of desirable posture

The major concern of the nurse in this respect is the prevention of contractures. Management begins immediately after admission. Although exercise regimes may be designed by the physiotherapist, it is essential for the nurse to understand the principles of positioning and exercising in order to initiate and provide continuity of care. In smaller hospitals nurses may have complete responsibility for this therapy.

If immediate care is not begun, the hemiplegic stroke patient will quickly adopt the typical stroke posture. Good positioning and support are necessary to maintain correct body alignment and prevent spasticity. Full-range passive exercises carried out three or four times a day help to prevent contractures. Even in the early stages the nurse should help to orientate the patient towards his affected half, by placing objects of interest on that side.

The role of the nurse here should extend to the patient's family and close friends, who should be taught and encouraged to participate in exercising and moving the patient.

Communication

Even in the acute stage of management of a stroke patient, the nurse needs to establish an effective level of communication with the patient. This should be kept simple but it must occur, otherwise the patient will remain isolated, bewildered and withdrawn. Lack of involvement of the patient in decision-making will lead to passivity and frustration. There may be confusion and disorientation in time and place, and the nurse can help to reorientate and provide clarity for a frightened patient. Wherever possible, relatives and friends should be encouraged to involve the patient in their conversations. A stroke victim does not revert to childhood: he is still an adult with adult emotions and desires. He should not be talked down to.

Restoration of function and rebuilding a productive life

After the early acute stage of illness, the stroke patient enters a prolonged period of regaining independence. The role of the nurse in providing continuity and consistency of therapy is vital.

Posture and mobility

A large portion of nursing time is devoted to helping the stroke patient initiate and control changes in posture associated with activities of living. Achievement depends on careful assessment of the patient's degree of motor, sensory and intellectual loss, and the skilled team planning of a therapy programme. Specific instruction for exercise regimes will be provided by the physiotherapist, with whom the nurse will work in close co-operation in mobilising the stroke patient. Improving mobility is the key to pressure sore prevention. Thought should be given to the patient's environment: there should be a non-slip floor, uncluttered by low-level obstructions, and furniture should be solid and carefully positioned to act as support and handrail. Chairs should give the necessary spinal support and allow the patient to place both feet squarely on the floor. Adjustable-height beds should be used and may be fitted with a detachable cot-side to act as a grab rail and provide a sense of security. A monkey pole over the head of the bed may encourage mobility and a sense of independence. The nurse should make full use of hoists and other aids to lifting, especially with severely disabled or very heavy stroke patients. The use of bath seats, rails and raised lavatory seats should be encouraged so that the patient's safety and sense of increasing freedom is maximised.

Eating and drinking

The nurse needs to assess the patient's nutritional requirements and take account of particular likes and dislikes. In addition, difficulties of chewing, swallowing and the mechanics of feeding may be overcome by thoughtful nursing and the careful use of aids. In the early stages of rehabilitation, the nurse may need to feed the patient. This often slow process should be an unhurried and comfortable one for both parties. Non-slip mats, plate guards and specially designed eating implements and containers are available, and should be used wherever appropriate and acceptable to the patient. The social aspect of eating should be encouraged.

A major factor in encouraging adequate eating and drinking is time. Meals should never be rushed and simple intervention, such as keeping food warm between courses, will be greatly appreciated. Mealtimes should be a pleasure, occasions to be enjoyed rather than dreaded and endured.

Elimination

The problems of urinary incontinence and constipation are not uncommon after stroke, and their successful management will do much to improve the patient's quality of life both personally and socially.

The control of micturition demands a positive attitude from the nurse. Full assessment of micturition pattern, including episodes of incontinence, is necessary before a retraining programme can begin. There is little hope of success in controlling incontinence unless lavatories or commodes are easily accessible, private, warm, clean and safe. Raised toilet seats, or commodes that are firm and secure, are more likely to encourage a relaxed emotional state where voiding will occur at the right time and in the right place. Teetering on a bedpan will do little to encourage urine flow.

For patients with persistent incontinence or for those in whom rehabilitation is incomplete, incontinence pads and pants can be used successfully. These pads should be the sort that keep the patient's urine from the skin. Condom sheath drainage, or dribble pouches may be considered for male patients. An indwelling catheter should be used only as a last resort. In such cases a closed drainage system must be used, so that the risk of urinary tract infection is minimised. Various clothing aids are now available to hold the drainage bag conveniently out of sight, to help maintain the patient's dignity.

For bowel retraining, a full assessment of normal bowel and dietary habits and mobility function is necessary. To begin with, it may be necessary to evacuate the rectum by use of an enema. Thereafter, management should be aimed at regular evacuation of soft faeces. A combination of diet, improving mobility and judicious use of safe laxatives will usually be successful.

Personal hygiene and dressing

Mobility difficulties, and sensory and emotional disturbances are likely to influence the patient's personal hygiene. The ability to wash, shave and take a bath or a shower is an important confidence booster.

Hoists, bath boards and stools, handrails, correct height wash basins should all be considered in order to provide safe and secure conditions for hygiene activities. For the hemiplegic patient, soap on a string, flannel mittens and long-handled brushes are aids to independence at bath time. Facial shaving for men can usually be accomplished independently. Care of hair and nails, and application of cosmetics may demand the assistance of the nurse or other carer: specially adapted implements, e.g. nail files, are available.

Clothing for the stroke patient often needs to be adapted to assist one-handed dressing and undressing. The actual activity of dressing and undressing will normally be taught by the occupational therapist but, once again, the nurse provides the continuity of care and encouragement.

Communication

There is probably no aspect of disability following a stroke that is more devastating than the disruption of speech. Some stroke patients will become and remain isolated as a result of gross language disturbance. Support for the patient and his family should begin immediately, whether at home or in hospital. The speech therapist provides the programme, but the nurses and relatives will need to provide constant stimulation and exercises. Group therapy sessions may be arranged but the one-to-one practice sessions for speech, reading and recognising, and writing, demand time and devoted attention, which should continue long after the patient has been discharged from the care of the health service.

Social, leisure and religious activities

These aspects of living are important in the rehabilitation of the stroke patient. The nurse can be the organiser for a wide range of social and recreational activities. Special events should be recognised and celebrated to act as a stimulus. The patients may be assisted to indulge in a variety of games that help in therapy as well as providing a social focus. The stroke patient may be able to continue a hobby, such as gardening or baking while he is recovering: this is particularly important if he is cared for at home. Improvisations and creative alterations to the institutional environment need not be costly or overwhelming but may stimulate the stroke patient to achieve a much-desired recreational goal, for example tomatoes could be grown on windowsills. Nurses and other carers may organise outings and visits for interest, shopping, family parties, etc.

The need for close personal relationships does not disappear when a patient has had a stroke. The nurse should become skilled to provide sexual counselling to stroke patients when required and should ensure a quiet, private place for stroke patients and their partners to be alone and intimate.

Finally, as with any other patient, spiritual activity and contact with spiritual advisers should be maintained. The role of the nurse in spiritual comfort is one of facilitator and provider of resources rather than being personally involved.

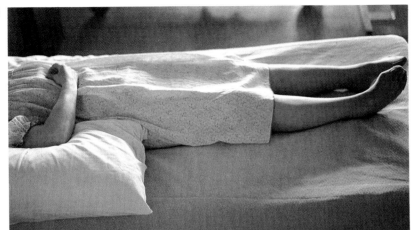

259 Hemiplegic posture (right-sided). The leg is in extension, the foot in plantar flexion, the arm pronated and flexed across the chest.

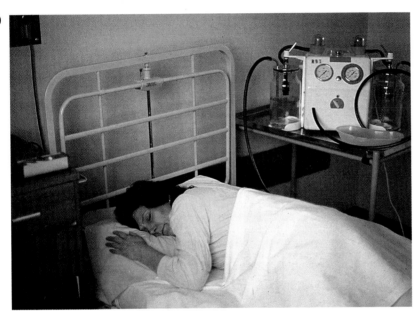

260 Unconscious patient being nursed on the side with suction and resuscitative equipment nearby.

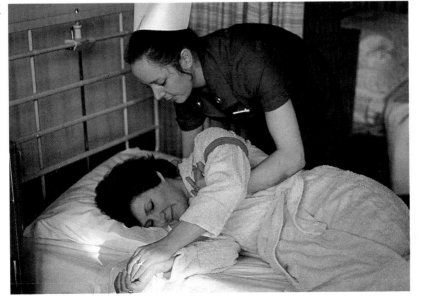

261 Moving a patient on to her side — correcting at the shoulder girdle. Hold the front of the underneath shoulder so that the nurse's forearm supports the head. With the other arm, hold the front of the affected shoulder. Move the patient's head and shoulder backwards so that the back is straight. The upper shoulder should be tipped slightly forward.

262 Sitting up in bed. The nurse approaches the patient from the affected side. She puts her left arm through the patient's arm as shown and grasps beneath the thigh. The patient braces her sound heel and the right hand on the bed and the nurse lifts her up. More disabled patients can be lifted by two nurses, one on either side.

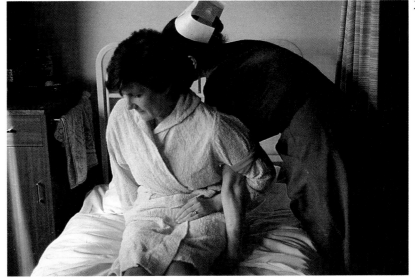

263 The stroke patient is now sitting up. Note the emergency call button lying close to the patient's unaffected hand and suction equipment in the background.

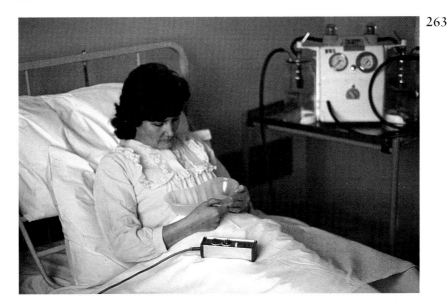

264 To sit up on the edge of the bed from a lying position, the patient first rolls on to her affected side. Then the legs are swung over the edge of the bed followed by taking the weight through the affected forearm and pushing up with the sound hand.

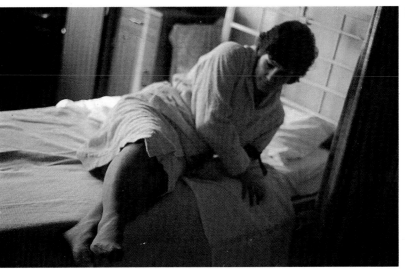

265

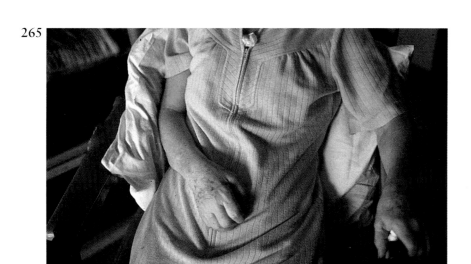

265 The paralysed right arm is slightly flexed at the elbow, which is supported with a soft pillow.

266

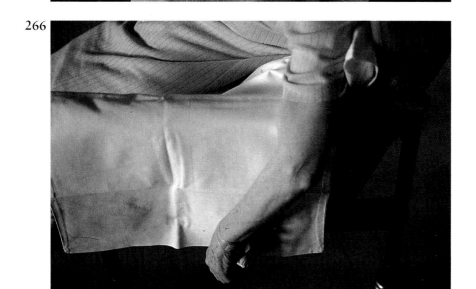

266 The paralysed arm is hanging over the side of the chair. This is a dangerous situation and indicates poor nursing. The patient is at risk from developing dislocation of the shoulder joint.

267

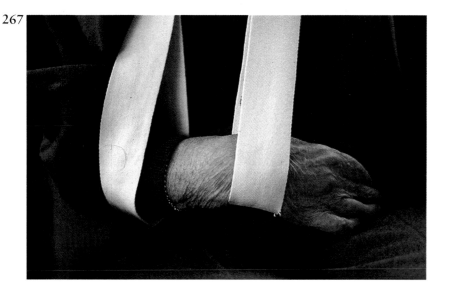

267 An arm with flaccid paralysis and painful shoulder may be supported by a sling.

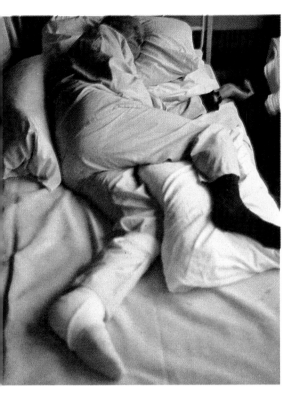

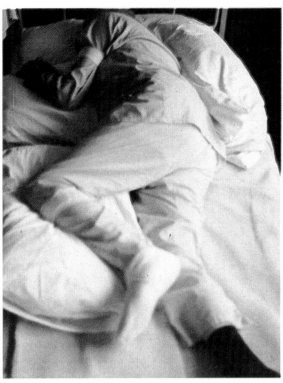

268 Lying on the affected side with shoulder well forward and elbow straight. The affected hip is as straight as possible. The sound leg is well forward and supported on a pillow.

269 Lying on the sound side with the affected shoulder well forward. The affected hip is forward with hip and knee bent and supported on a pillow.

270 Lying on the back. The patient should try to avoid this position. The head is turned to the affected side and the affected arm, trunk and hip are supported on a pillow.

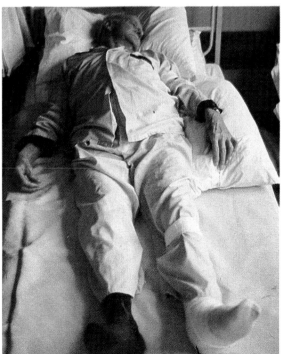

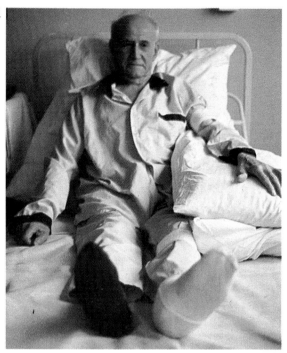

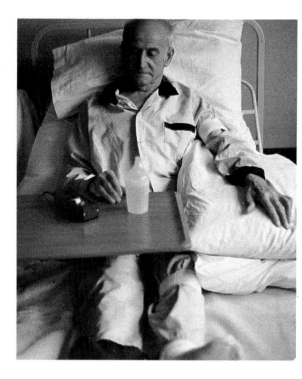

271 Sitting up in bed with trunk as upright as possible. The affected shoulder is well forward and the arm is supported on a cushion. The weight is placed equally on both hips and the legs are straight out.

272 Sitting up in bed with a table at the front.

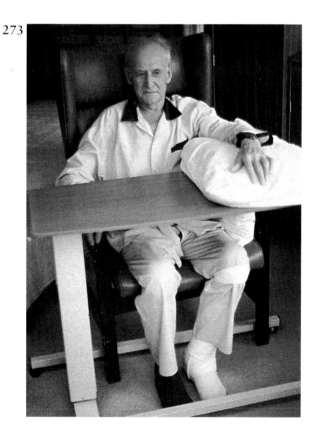

273 Sitting up in a chair with the affected shoulder well forward, the arm on a pillow and feet flat on the floor.

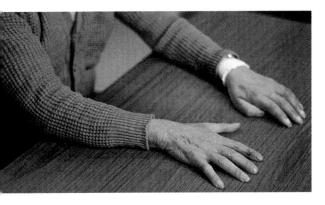

274 **Sitting at table with both forearms on the surface and hands flat with palms touching the table.** Both arms should look and feel the same.

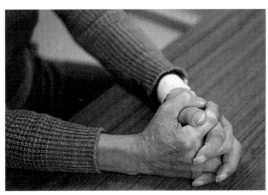

275 **Clasping hands with fingers interlocked** helps to maintain body symmetry. It keeps the affected arm in sight and prevents spasticity in the hand.

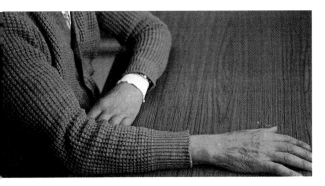

276 **Elbow bending.** The affected and sound arm should be exercised whilst sitting at the table. Elbow bending is done with both elbows supported on the table.

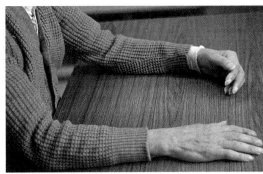

277 **Turning the hand over** is another useful exercise.

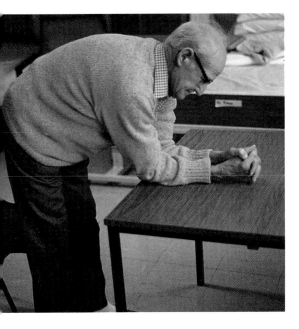

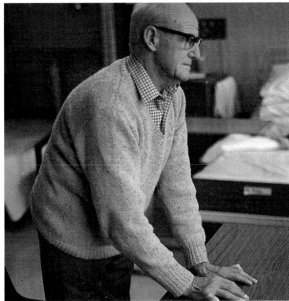

278 a) and b) **Standing from sitting at table.** The hands should be clasped supported on the table. Slowly the patient leans forward and lifts his trunk, supporting the weight on the forearms. Then he pushes up with his arms to straighten the body.

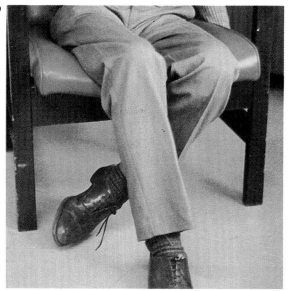

279 In the absence of adequate rehabilitation, the hemiplegic left leg will adopt the position shown here. This will promote spasticity and make subsequent mobilisation difficult.

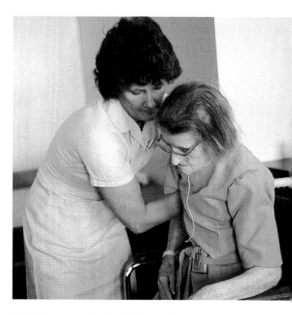

280 Wrong method of helping the patient to stand. Never pull by the arms or shoulders.

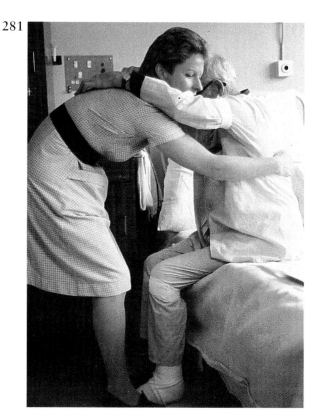

281 Helping the patient to stand. The patient clasps his hands behind the nurse who blocks the patient's knees and feet. The patient rocks forward and with the aid of momentum stands up slowly. If the patient is to be transferred then swivel the patient around to the chair or commode.

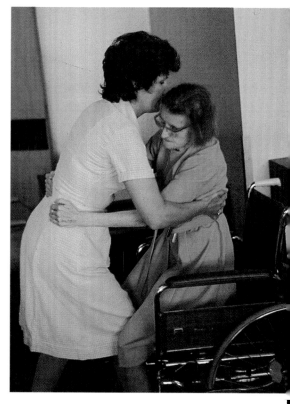

282 A more disabled patient with stiff shoulders may be assisted to stand and transfer as shown here.

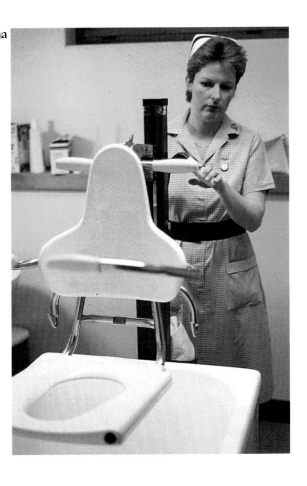

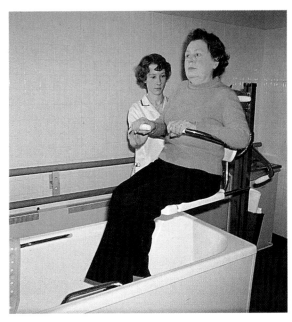

283 a) and b) **Hoists** should be used for lifting and moving heavy and severely disabled patients.

284 **A toilet with hand rails or frame** is a useful aid for patients with hemiplegia. It gives the patient confidence and makes the nursing easier.

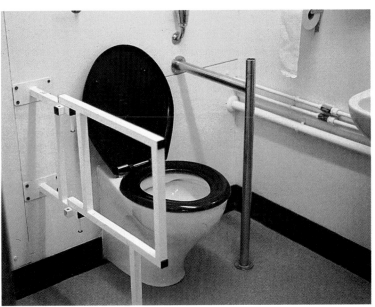

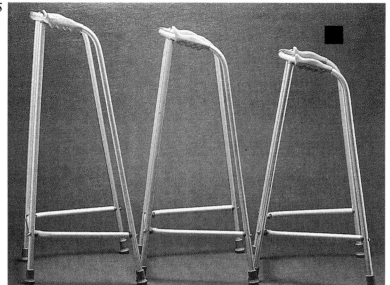

285 Walking frames are particularly useful for some elderly stroke patients.

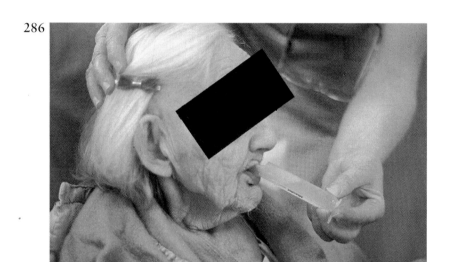

286 Correct feeding of the patient with deglutition problems is an important part of nursing care. Here the nurse is using a specially designed feeder for giving small quantities of liquids.

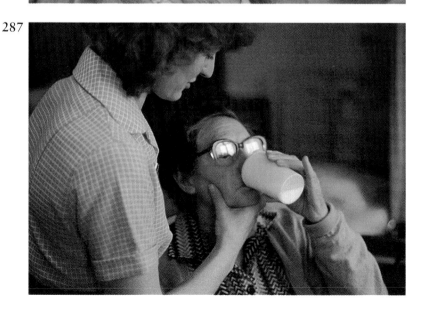

287 Assisted drinking by using the jaw grip to open and close the patient's mouth.

288 Poor oral hygiene can result in secondary infection with *Candida*.

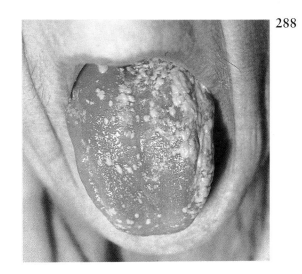

289 Ill-fitting dentures can cause problems after a stroke, because of the alteration of the oral anatomy.

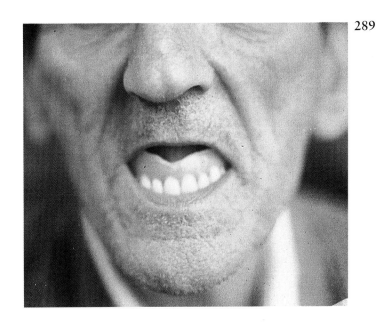

290 Incorrect handling of the patient in the early stages will give rise to later complications, such as a spastic hemiplegic hand.

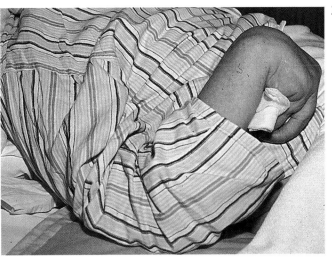

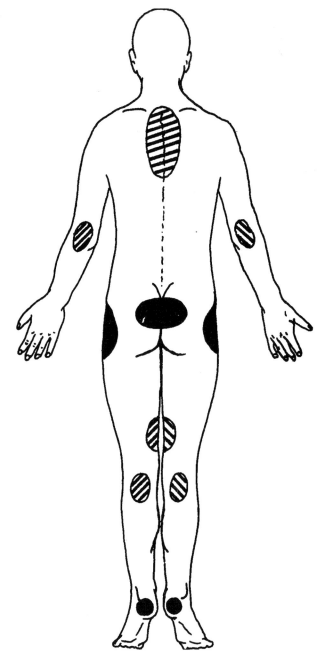

291 Areas susceptible to pressure sores — especially the sacrum, hips and heels.

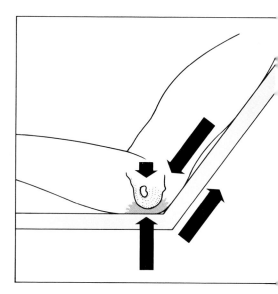

292 Compression and shearing forces involved in producing a pressure sore.

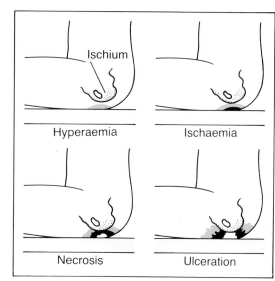

Ischium

Hyperaemia

Ischaemia

Necrosis

Ulceration

293 Stages in the development of a pressure sore.

294 Beginnings of a pressure sore. There is hyperaemia but the skin is intact.

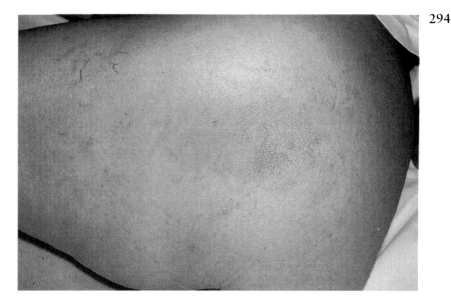

295 A large pressure sore with a dry necrotic scab.

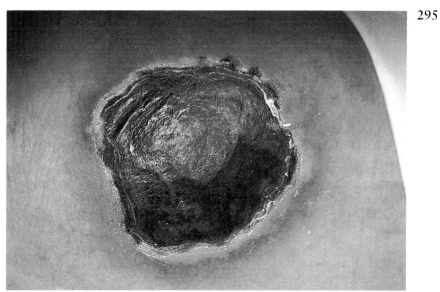

296 Pressure sore: deep, but with healing edges.

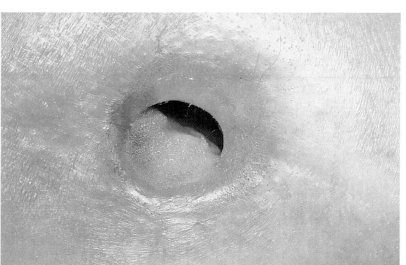

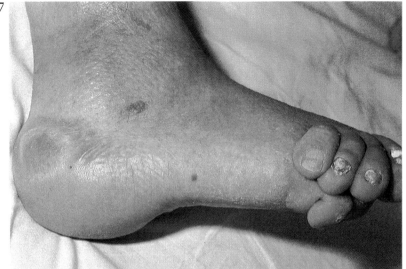

297 Early heel sore.

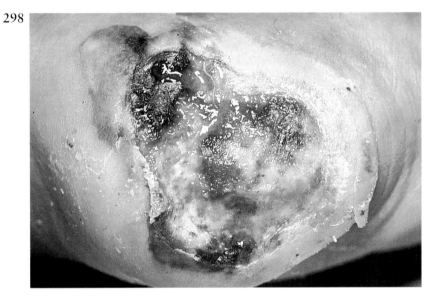

298 An advanced heel sore with much necrosis and secondary infection.

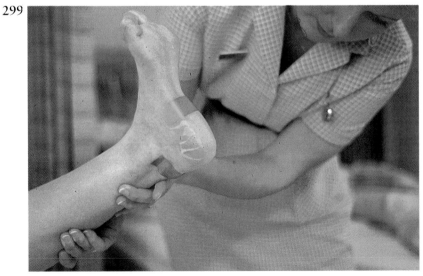

299 Nurse applying a protective heel dressing to a patient at risk.

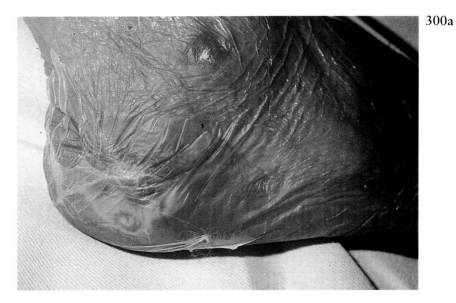

300a

300 a) and b) **Early heel sores** protected with a clear plastic dressing.

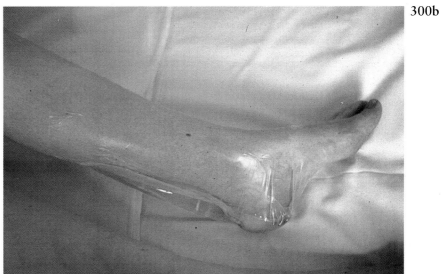

300b

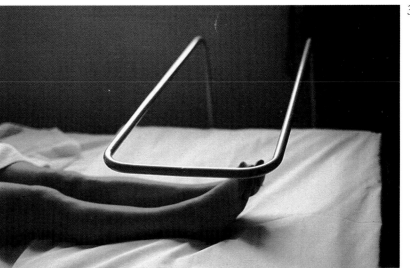

301

301 **A bed cradle** should be used to protect the feet.

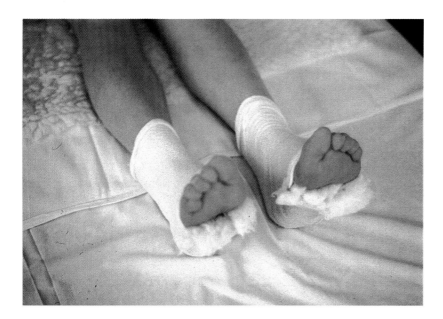

302 **Woollen heel pads** to protect the heels.

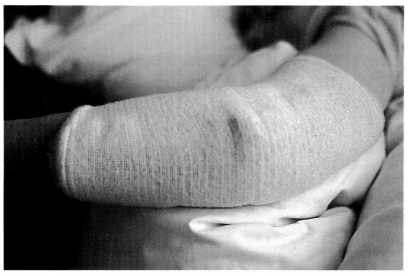

303 **A soft dressing over the hemiplegic elbow** to protect against a pressure sore.

304

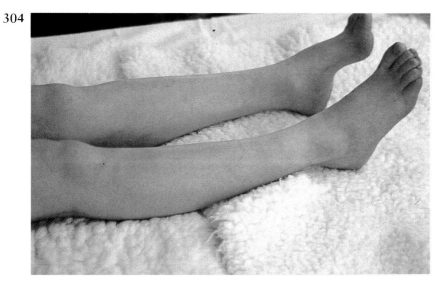

304 **Sheepskin** is useful in preventing pressure sores.

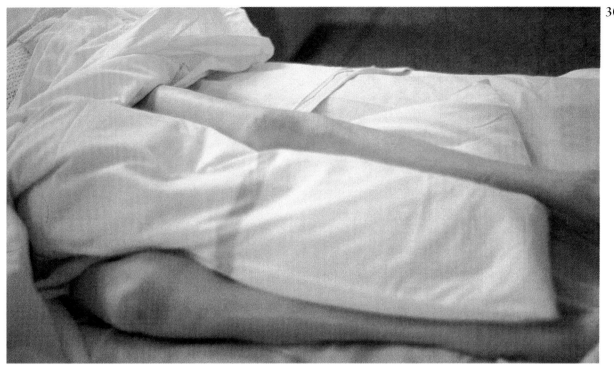

305 **A soft pillow** between the legs will protect the knees from developing pressure sores.

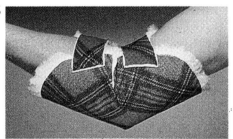
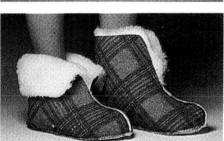
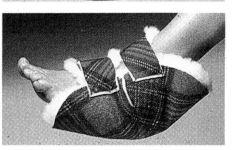

306 **Synthetic fleece protection.** The joint pads can be used to protect both elbows and heels.

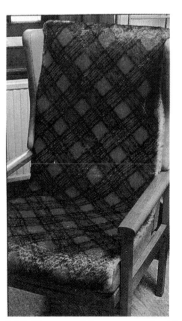
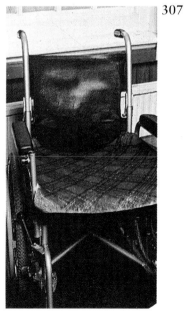

307 **Fleece cushions** are a valuable aid in nursing immobile hemiplegic patients who may be at risk from developing pressure sores.

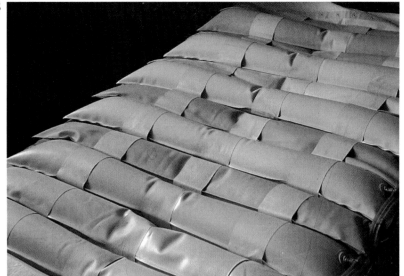

308 A large-celled alternating pressure mattress for prevention of pressure sores (ripple mattress).

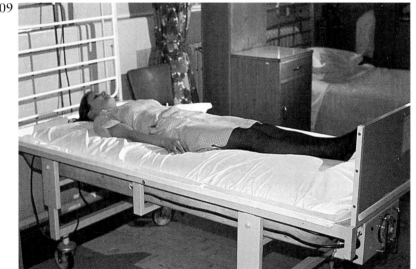

309 Water beds are used for both prevention and treatment of pressure sores. Elderly patients may not find them very comfortable and some complain of 'sea-sickness'.

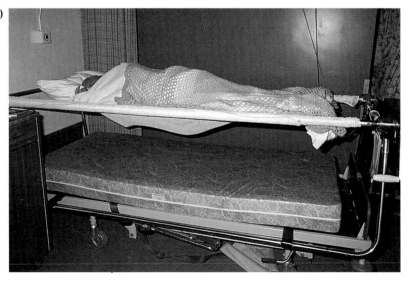

310 Net suspension bed is useful in lightening the nursing load and turning heavy patients in the prevention and treatment of pressure sores.

311 Neurological control of the bladder. In stroke the urinary incontinence results from a lesion in the higher cerebral centres.

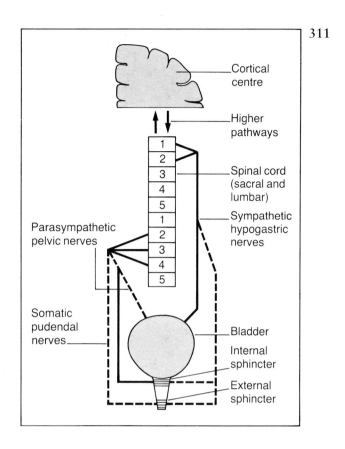

Cortical centre

Higher pathways

Spinal cord (sacral and lumbar)

Sympathetic hypogastric nerves

Parasympathetic pelvic nerves

Somatic pudendal nerves

Bladder

Internal sphincter

External sphincter

312 Rash caused by urinary incontinence.

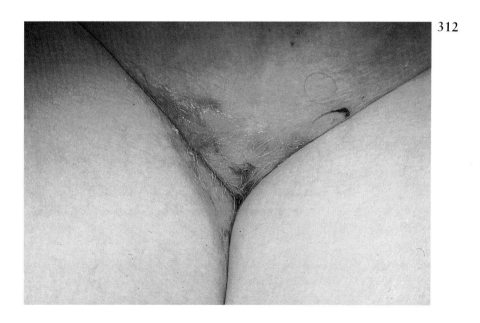

313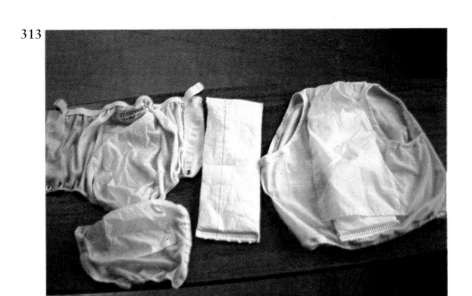

313 Marsupial pads and pants for managing incontinence in female patients.

314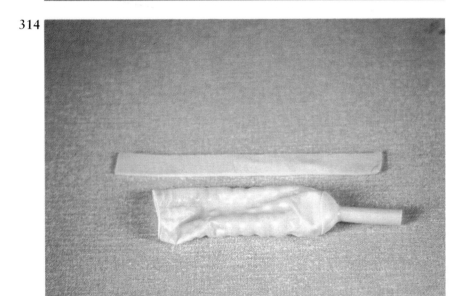

314 The condom urinary incontinence sheath is held to the penis by an internal adhesive fixature or an external compression strap. This is connected to a drainage bag. Sheaths are unsuitable for men who have a retracted penis.

315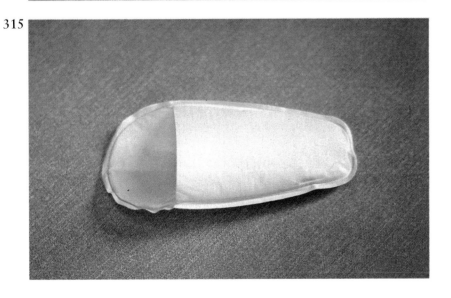

315 A dribble pouch is worn under the trousers, into which the penis fits. Absorbent material within the pouch will cope with up to 50 ml of urine.

316 Catheterisation should be the last resort in management of incontinence. A wide choice of different materials, shaft diameter, length and balloon sizes is available. The drainage should be unobtrusive and worn on the body, under the clothes, not on full view as shown here.

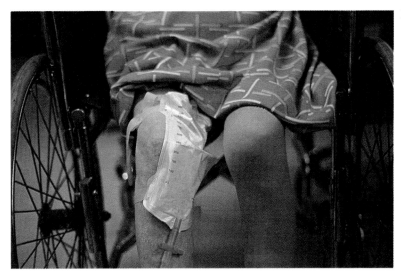

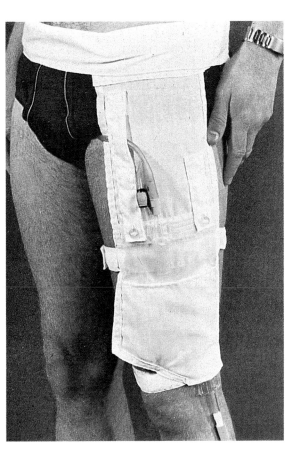

317 A closed urinary drainage system is both dignified and easy to manage.

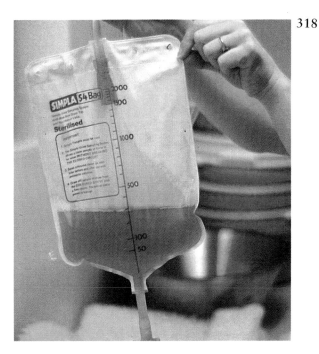

318 Urinary tract infection is a common problem in patients who have indwelling catheters. Frequent bladder washouts, adequate fluid intake and correct use of antibiotics are essential. Cloudy urine is caused by debris shed from the bladder.

319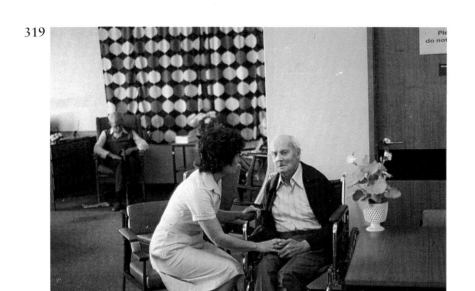

319 A rehabilitation ward must have a pleasant atmosphere. The day room should be spacious and uncrowded for successful rehabilitation. Note the nurse approaching the patient from the hemiplegic side.

320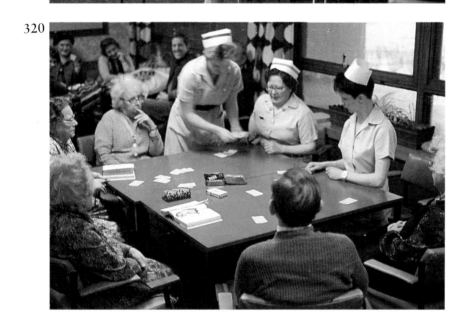

320 Placing a group of stroke patients together is advantageous. Here the nurses have joined the patients in playing a game. This generates an optimistic atmosphere both in the patients and the staff.

REHABILITATION

Pauline Watson and Janice Corlett

Bobath method: a form of rehabilitation in which an attempt is made to change abnormal patterns of posture and movements by using 'key points' of control. The principles of the Bobath method are used in this chapter.

Rehabilitation is an attempt to restore the patient to the maximum possible level of ability. It is essential to view the patient as a whole and be fully aware of the associated conditions and the complications of a stroke. The Bobath principles of stroke rehabilitation are gaining increasing popularity and are now practised widely, especially in the wards and units for stroke patients. However, in the elderly, pure Bobath method may be difficult to apply. It is often necessary to make adjustments. Mechanical aids such as tripods, walking frames and calipers may have to be used.

There are, of course, other methods of stroke rehabilitation. The effectiveness of each method, to a large extent, depends upon the criteria used for selecting patients and the enthusiasm of the therapist. The Brunnström training programme is based on the use of reflex movements known as associated reactions. The aim here is to promote the reflex mechanisms and try to help the patient develop cortical control over them. An attempt is made to improve function through positioning and associated reflexes.

Sensory loss and hemiplegia

Physiotherapy and occupational therapy

In the days following a stroke the patient may be able to do very little for himself. He needs sensory input to inform him of his body's position in order to perform a controlled movement successfully. If his sensation is impaired, but not completely lost, he may feel as if his body has two separate halves that no longer work together. He may describe his affected limbs as feeling heavy and stiff. If sensation is lost on the affected side, the patient is likely to neglect that side. This neglect may be compounded by homonymous hemianopia — a visual disturbance where the patient is unable to see an object placed on his affected side.

In the early stages the patient will probably present with a lack of muscle tone in the hemiplegic limbs. As soon as he is able, he will shift his balance away from the affected side and learn to compensate by doing everything with the normal side only. If this is allowed to continue, he will learn only abnormal patterns of movement.

Spasticity. This is an abnormal increase of muscle tone with exaggerated tendon reflexes. Some degree of spasticity is found in almost every hemiplegic patient. It causes the sensation of stiffness, provides a resistance to movement and makes the limbs seem weak. When spasticity is present in the neck and trunk, it causes retraction of the shoulder girdle and hip. This in turn causes a pattern of flexion spasticity in the arm and extension spasticity in the leg. A slight degree of spasticity will not stop the patient from learning to move his affected side again. However, this movement will not be fully controlled and co-ordinated, and he may be unable to use his affected side to take part in functional tasks, such as opening jars, writing, and tying his shoe laces. At the other extreme, a strong degree of spasticity can rob the patient of movement on the affected side and fix it in such an abnormal position that being washed and dressed is difficult and painful, and even sitting in a chair may be uncomfortable.

Spasticity is influenced by the way the patient positions and moves his body. If he uses effort when moving, spasticity will be increased by what is known as an 'associated reaction'. Associated reactions are reflex movements, for example if the unaffected arm is flexed against resistance, the paretic arm will reflexly assume a flexed position. Strong emotional feelings will also increase spasticity, e.g. fear and anxiety, pain, anger and frustration.

Principles of treatment

Teach the patient a relaxed approach to treatment: if effort is reduced, there will be less spasticity. Encourage weight-bearing throughout the affected side as part of the process of gaining normal balance and minimizing the fear of falling. Weight-bearing through the joints provides sensory feedback, telling the patient where his limbs are and facilitating movement in the affected side.

Work against the spastic pattern, i.e. encourage positions and movements involving neck, trunk and upper limb extension, and lower limb flexion. The following illustrations demonstrate these techniques of treatment with regard to:

- Handling and positioning the patient in the early stages.
- Early control of spasticity and movement.
- Working for recovery in the upper limb.
- Working for standing and walking.
- Activities of daily living.
- Coping with complications.

Handling and positioning the patient in the early stages

On some of the illustrations the affected side is indicated by red bands.

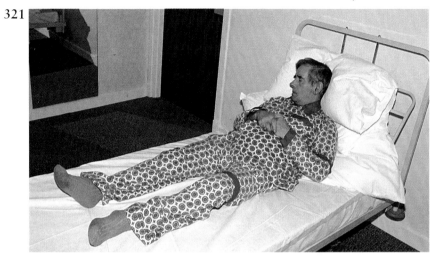

321 Typical position of the patient in bed — incorrect.

- Head turned away from the affected side
- Neck flexed
- Shoulder retracted
- Arm held protectively
- Hip retracted
- Leg rolled out to the side
- Foot pointing down

The risk of complications, such as neglect of the affected side, painful shoulder, spasticity and contractures, can be reduced by correct positioning of the patient.

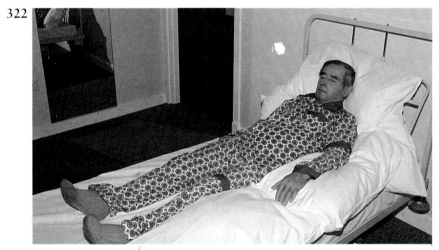

322 Correct position of the patient in bed.

- Head in midline
- Staggered pillows reducing neck flexion
- Pillow under the shoulder preventing retraction
- Arm fully supported in extension
- Hip re-positioned
- Pillow to prevent the leg rolling out

Lying on the back can increase spasticity: side-lying is preferable, especially on the affected side.

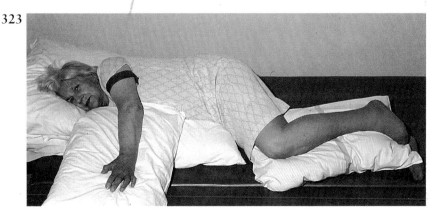

323 Side-lying — on the sound side.

- The affected arm should be brought well forward at right angles to the body, supported in extension by a pillow
- The leg should be flexed, supported by a pillow

Lying in one position for a long time may cause pressure sores and also encourages the patient to shuffle about, thereby destroying his good position.

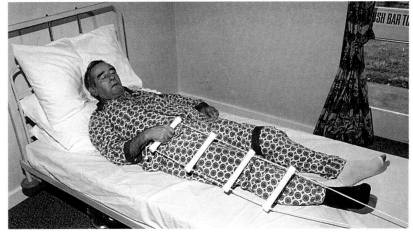

324 Sitting up in bed — harmful: the effort required to pull on the bed ladder causes increased spasticity on the affected side. Many patients with dense hemiplegia cannot use a bed ladder as one arm is completely paralysed.

325 Moving up the bed with a monkey pole — harmful: this requires even more effort than the bed ladder. Assisting the patient as illustrated will damage the shoulder.

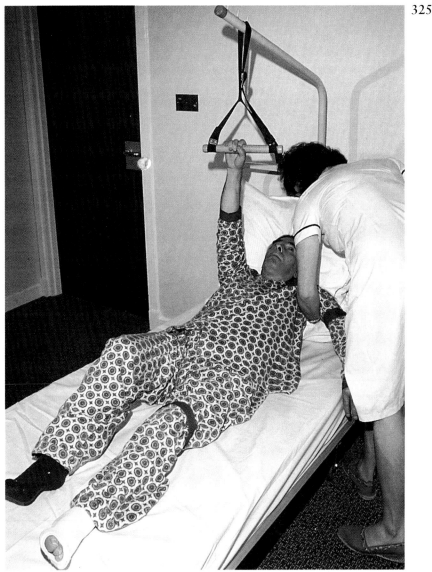

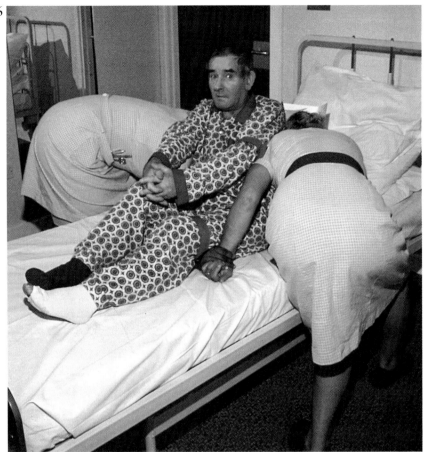

326

Moving up the bed can be too difficult a manoeuvre for the stroke patient to attempt in the early stages.

326 Moving up the bed — Australian lift. Safest method: requires no effort from the patient and avoids damage to the shoulder.

327

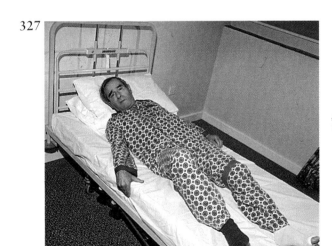

327 Rolling over in bed — harmful: the patient automatically tries to push or pull with his sound side. The effort required increases spasticity.

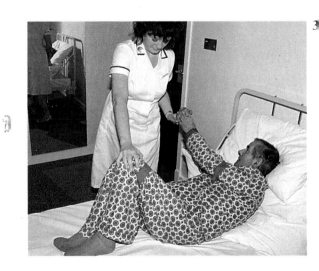

328 Rolling over in bed — starting position. With knees flexed, the patient turns his head, reaches right across with his arms, and his legs should automatically follow.

Getting out of bed on the affected side is more therapeutic, as weight-bearing stimulates awareness of the paralysed limbs.

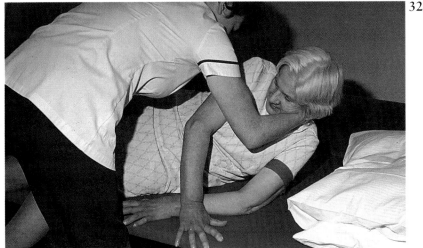

329 Getting out of bed. After rolling over and bringing the legs over the side of the bed, the patient learns to take weight through the affected arm while using the sound arm to push up into the sitting position, thereby reducing effort. For a long time the patient may need help to bring his legs out of bed.

330–332 Transferring from bed to wheelchair.

- The patient is brought to the edge of the bed
- His affected knee is supported
- His arms are placed around the lifter's waist
- His affected shoulder is supported to prevent damage
- Standing up is initiated by the patient leaning forwards

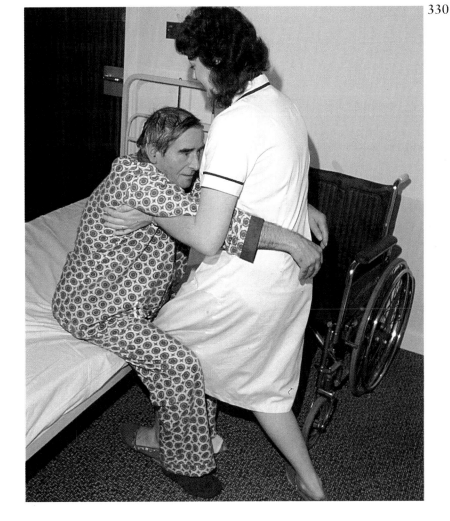

To minimize effort, the wheelchair should be placed at right angles and as close as possible to the patient before transferring.

331

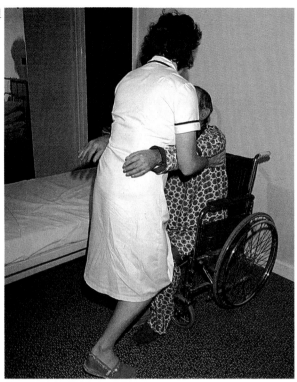

- The patient must not pull on the lifter
- The lifter turns the patient round
- The patient leans forward to sit

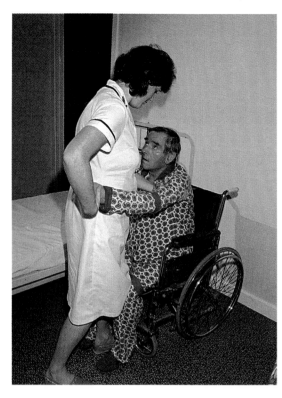

- Correctly positioned in the chair, the affected arm is carefully released and not allowed to drop

333

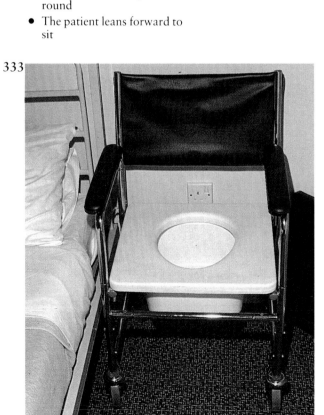

333 **Use of commode.** Getting into position to use a bedpan can require much effort. Transferring on to a commode is preferable.

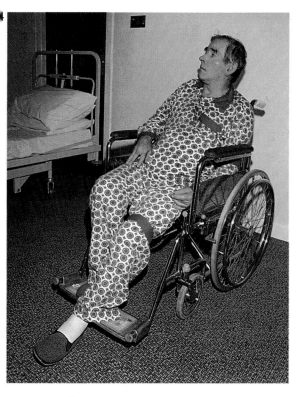

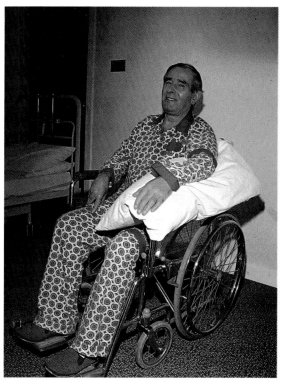

334 Typical sitting position — incorrect.

- Head turned away from the affected side
- Shoulder depressed and retracted
- Arm trapped and in flexion
- Hip retracted
- Leg extended and externally rotated
- No weight-bearing through affected heel

It is most important to encourage weight-bearing through the affected side from an early stage.

335 Correct sitting position.

- Attention drawn to the affected side
- Pillow supporting the shoulder in elevation and protraction
- Arm supported in extension
- Hip position corrected
- Leg flexed with hip, knee and ankle at 90°
- Weight-bearing through heel on footrest

In the early stages the patient will spend most of his time sitting down. It is important that a suitable armchair is chosen.

336 Typical easy chair — incorrect.

- Most body weight is going through the sacrum
- The patient is leaning back
- The patient is slumped with head supported
- Seat is too long, inhibiting knee flexion
- No weight-bearing through heel
- Chair too low to stand up without effort

Head support on a chair interferes with relearning head control. A reclining back interferes with learning balance, a tip-back chair being the worst example.

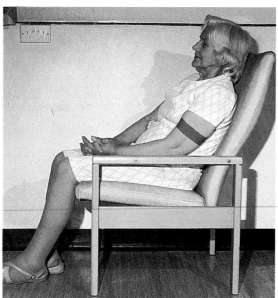

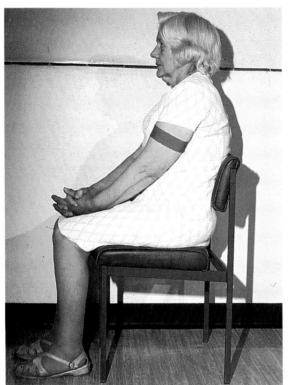

337

337 Correct shape of chair.

- Equal body weight through ischial tuberosities
- The patient is sitting upright
- The patient has responsibility for head control
- Hips, knees and ankles are at 90°
- Weight-bearing through the heel
- Choose correct height for standing up

It is good for the patient to learn to sit in a chair without arms, but this takes time and careful supervision. If the patient is to remain seated for any length of time a chair with more padding is essential for comfort.

A variety of methods can be used to raise an armchair or bed to a suitable height for the patient to sit correctly and stand up with minimal effort.

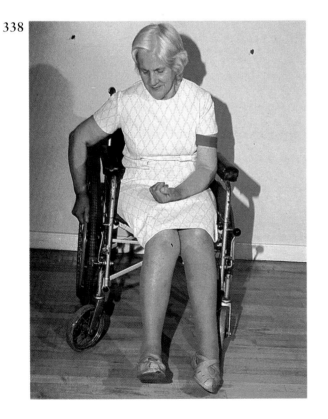

338

338 Associated reactions to effort. Increased spasticity in the form of flexion in the arm and extension in the leg.

Operating a wheelchair with the sound side requires a lot of effort and draws attention away from the affected side.

It is preferable for someone else to push the wheelchair in the early stages, and for the patient to concentrate on standing and walking as soon as he is ready.

Early control of spasticity and movement

The patient may be treated on the ward or in the physiotherapy and occupational therapy departments. Rehabilitation carried out by the nursing staff and relatives is important and therefore the physician in charge may prefer to continue rehabilitation on the ward. A stroke unit is ideal, but most hospitals do not have one.

The physiotherapist works with the patient to achieve control of movement combined with inhibition of spasticity.

339 Trunk rotation. The physiotherapist passively rotates the trunk to achieve elongation in the affected side, inhibiting spasticity. Eventually, the patient is taught actively to rotate his trunk himself.

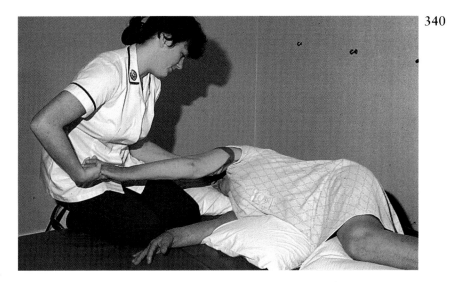

339

340 Control of the shoulder. The patient is reaching forward with assistance. Reaching forward (protraction) is the opposite to the spastic pattern (retraction). Work begins on the shoulder as it tends to recover before the rest of the arm.

340

341 Inhibitory position of the arm. When attempting to gain control of the hip the sound arm moves the affected arm into a position of extension to inhibit any associated reaction to effort.

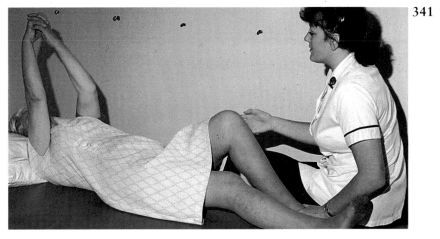

341

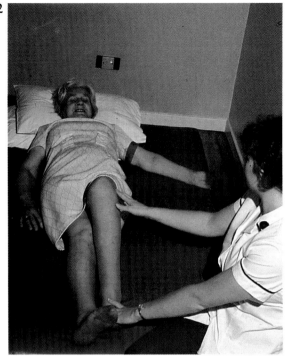

342 Alternative inhibitory position of arm. The arm is placed in the opposite position to that of spasticity.

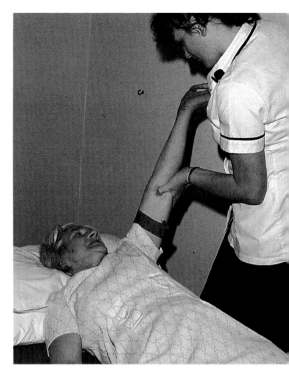

343 Work on the shoulder girdle. The physiotherapist is helping the patient to gain protraction of the shoulde

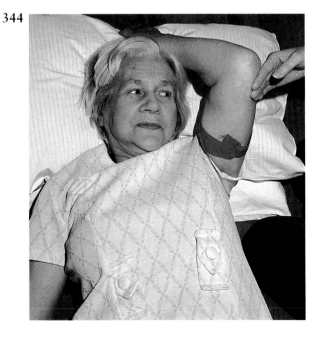

344 Elbow extension. The patient is attempting a selective movement — elbow extension — without shoulder movement.

Having begun by working on the trunk, followe by the shoulder girdle, treatment progresses to th elbow, the wrist and finally the hand as recover takes place. Similar progression occurs in th lower limb.

Working for recovery in the upper limb

As well as being able to perform a movement in the physiotherapy department, it is important that the patient can use his skills during the rest of his day. The occupational therapist introduces activities that reinforce normal movement patterns, while providing the satisfaction of being able to do something successfully. Activities that appeal to the patient should always be chosen in order to gain his maximum co-operation. However, care must be taken to ensure that he is always practising the correct movements and not getting side-tracked by the task itself.

Excessive effort should be avoided and heavy activities should be used only if the patient has sufficient control to work without associated reactions of increased spasticity.

345 Weight-bearing through the forearm. The physiotherapist can begin teaching weight-bearing through the forearm, to inhibit spasticity and stimulate sensory feedback.

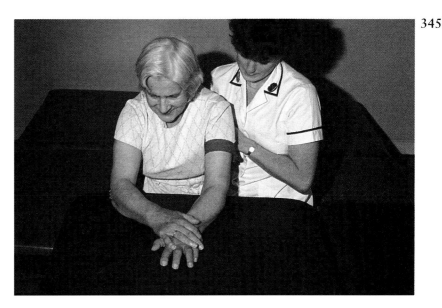

345

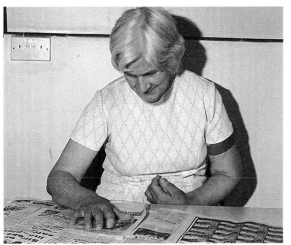

346 Typical position when sitting at a table. Harmful: attention is directed towards the sound side, the affected hip and shoulder are retracted, the arm flexed and spastic.

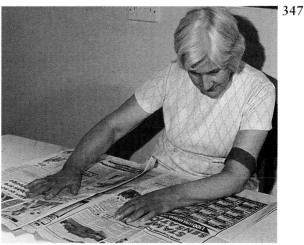

347

347 Weight-bearing while reading. Attention is equally divided between both sides. Weight-bearing is inhibiting spasticity.

If the patient sits at a table of the correct height during the day, he will eventually be able to get into a weight-bearing position independently to read, write letters, etc.

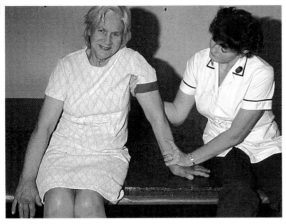

348 Weight-bearing through the extended arm. Most patients sit with more weight on their sound side. Here the physiotherapist is encouraging the patient to transfer body weight towards the affected side both through the arm and the pelvis.

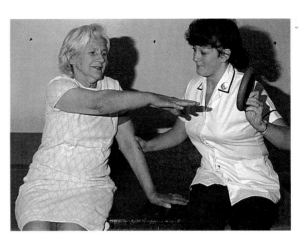

349 Trunk rotation. The patient is weight-bearing and rotating the trunk by reaching across to the affected side.

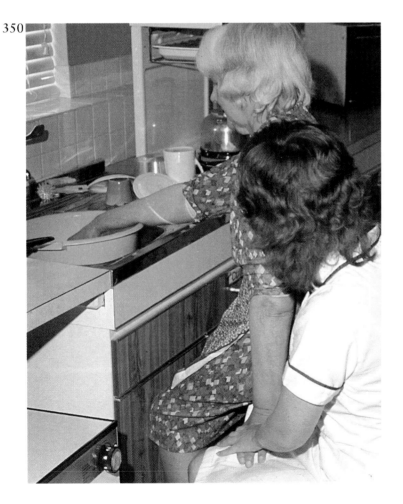

350 Weight-bearing during functional activity. The occupational therapist is reinforcing weight-bearing to inhibit spasticity while the patient is sitting to wash up.

351 Inhibition of spasticity while sitting. If flexor spasticity is very strong and the patient cannot maintain the arm in extension at the side, it can be moved backwards in full external rotation of the shoulder.

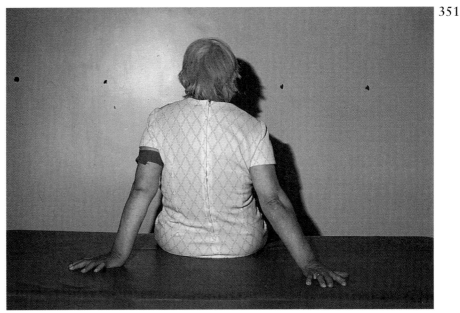

352 Inhibition of spasticity while standing. Note that in sitting and standing the sound arm should be placed in the same position as the affected arm to keep the shoulders level.

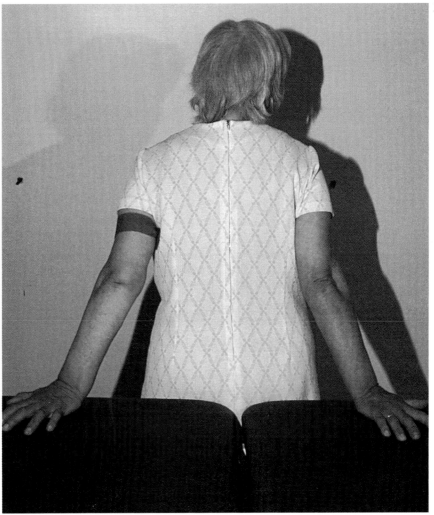

353

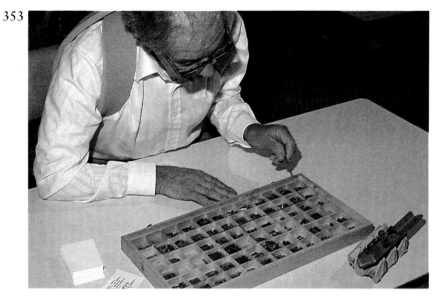

353 Weight-bearing activity.
In the early stages, when the patient has no functional control of movement, activities such as setting up printing can be carried out, emphasizing correct weight-bearing.

354

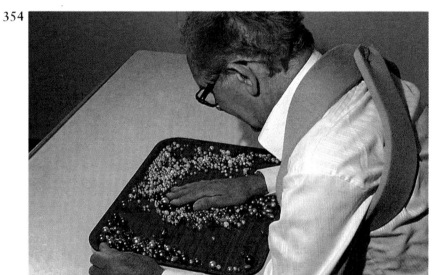

354 Sensory input. Working with different textures and shapes helps to provide tactile input.

355

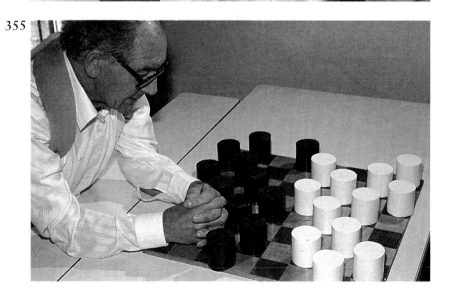

355 Bilateral activities. The sound arm assists the affected arm to play draughts, encouraging leaning forward with trunk extension, shoulder protraction and elbow extension while maintaining sitting balance.

356 Gross movement. The patient practises protraction of the shoulder and extension of the elbow going forwards, and returning backwards. The polishing block slides easily on the board cutting down resistance to movement.

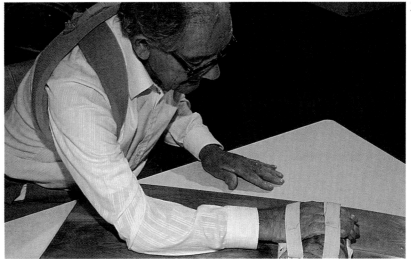

357 Control. The patient needs to push the ball only gently as both ball and skittles are very light. He must avoid jerky movements and turning his arm into a flexor spasticity position.

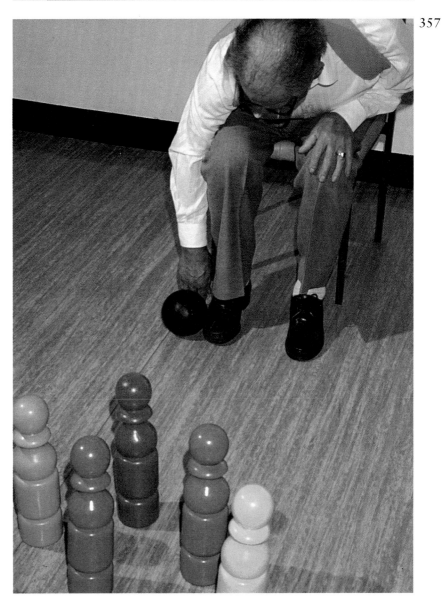

358

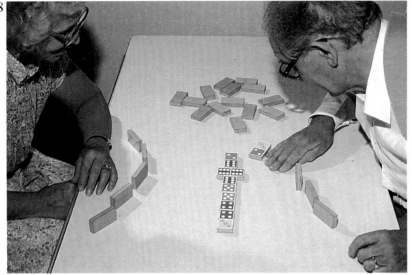

358 Selective movement. The elbow is resting on the table to support the weight of the arm. The patient works on selective movements of elbow and shoulder to place the dominoes.

359

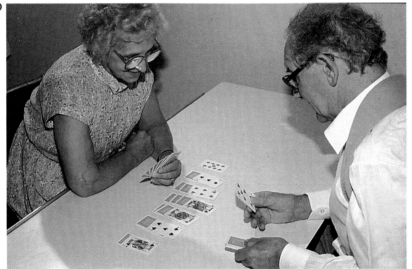

359 Synchronized control. The patient has to grip the card, turn it into supination, combine movements of shoulder and elbow to place it. then release grip. If spasticity increased, the patient would fail.

360

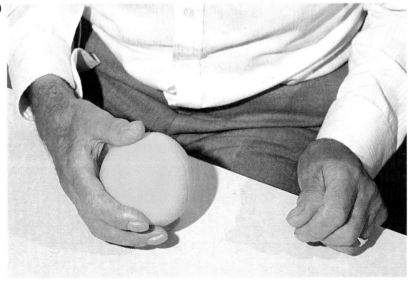

360 Squeezing a ball. Harmful: it must be remembered that the aid is to teach control, concentrating on the opposite to the spastic pattern. Squeezing a ball requires flexion with effort; this will increase spasticity.

If the patient's relatives can be involved they should be encouraged to continue treatment at home, but they will need to be instructed how to do this on the ward first.

Working for standing and walking

As well as working for selective movement of the lower limb, it is important to practise the correct movement patterns for standing up and walking.

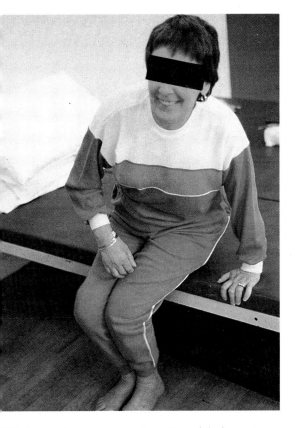

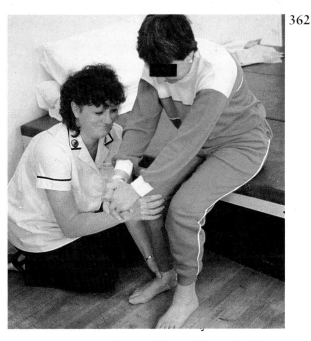

362 Correct pattern for standing up. The patient is encouraged to maintain symmetry when standing up from sitting. Note how she is encouraged to bear weight through the affected side by placing the affected foot behind.

361 Instinctive way to stand up. Harmful: the patient transfers her weight to the sound side and pushes extremely hard through the sound arm and leg. There is no weight on the affected side, so no inhibition of the associated reaction.

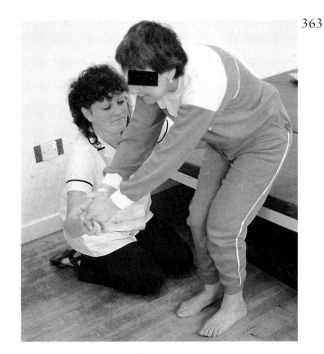

363 She is then encouraged to lean well forward over her feet and keep her weight evenly distributed through both sides. Most stroke patients will automatically take more weight through the sound side, and this is the case with this particular patient.

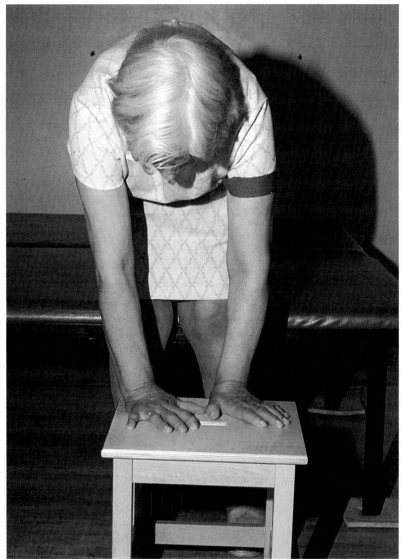

364

364 Leaning forward to stand. The patient may need encouragement to lean far enough forward to stand up successfully. Weight-bearing on a stool can help.

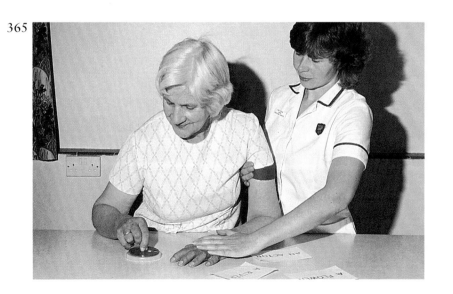

365

365 Standing balance. In the early stages standing can be very frightening. Weight-bearing through the forearm on a high table can inhibit any associated reaction of spasticity and build up confidence. The occupational therapist can introduce an activity such as a quiz game, which requires little physical effort.

6

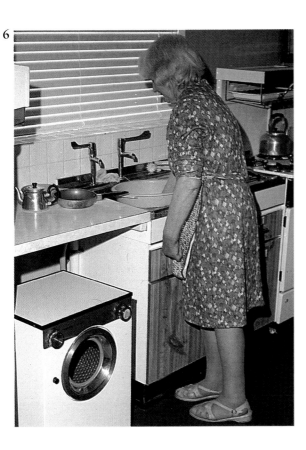

366 Typical standing position. Harmful: the patient approached the sink leaving the affected side behind. No weight, therefore no inhibition, on the affected side. The effort of washing-up causes visible flexor spasticity in the wrist and fingers.

367

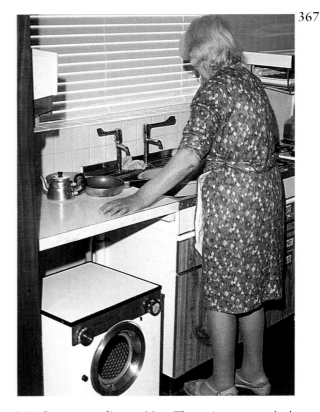

367 Correct standing position. The patient approached the sink properly and has equal weight through both sides. There is a little weight-bearing through the affected arm and spasticity is inhibited.

8

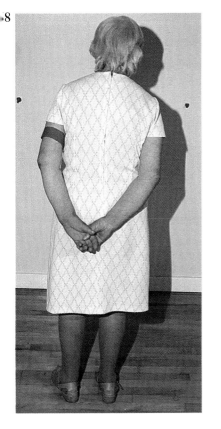

368 Typical weight-bearing in standing. Harmful: most of the weight is on the sound side. The patient needs to take equal weight through both legs to inhibit spasticity and achieve a good walking pattern.

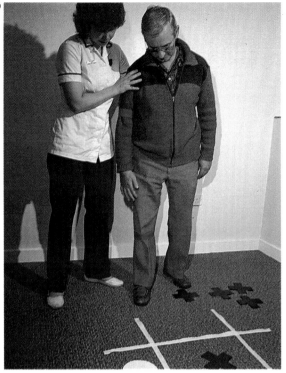

369

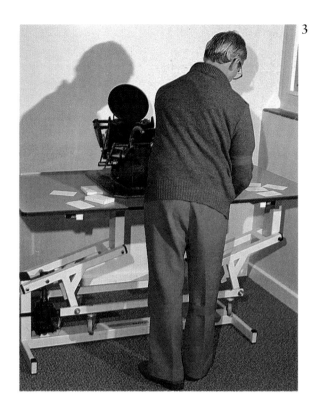

3

369 Weight-bearing during an activity. The occupational therapist plays floor noughts and crosses with the patient. He must bear weight through his affected leg while moving the pieces with his sound leg.

370 Weight transference in standing. The occupational therapist has placed cards to be printed on the sound side, and room for the finished cards on the affected side. This encourages the patient to reach from side to side, achieving trunk rotation and transference of weight from one foot to the other.

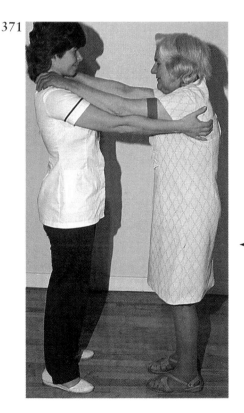

371

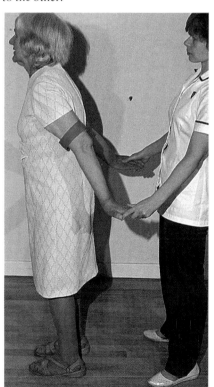

3

Walking should begin with assistance from the therapist and ideally without letting the patient use any form of walking aid. However, many elderly patients will feel more confident and safe with an aid such as a walking frame.

◀ **371 Assisted walking.** The therapist is maintaining shoulder protraction to inhibit spasticity, which may increase with the effort and anxiety of early walking.

372 An alternative method of inhibition. ▶

Some patients, particularly the elderly, will not achieve independence without a walking aid, e.g. a walking stick, tripod or Zimmer frame.

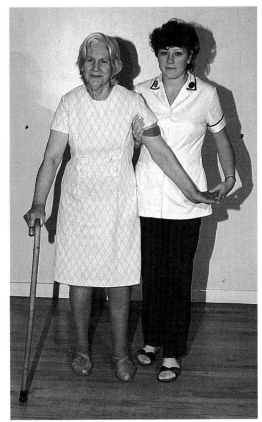

373

373 Walking with a stick. The walking stick is purposely too long so that it can be used purely as an aid to balance, the patient maintaining equal weight-bearing and symmetry. If spasticity increases, the therapist can inhibit it by maintaining the arm in extension.

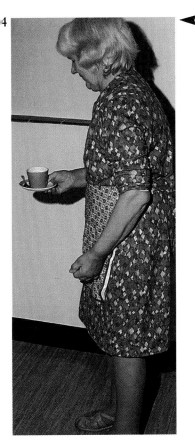

374 Carrying. Harmful: attempting to walk and carry a cup of tea requires effort and concentration. Visible flexor spasticity is the result.

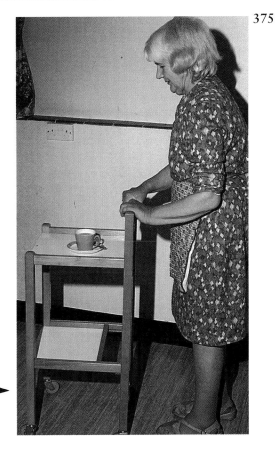

375

375 Trolley. The occupational therapist can provide a trolley to make it easier to carry things.

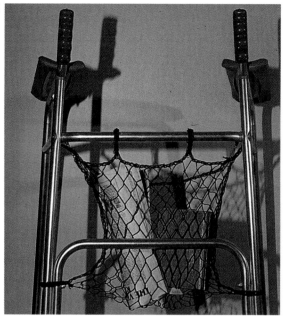

376 Net bag. If the patient has to use a rollator frame, the occupational therapist can provide a net bag to fit on to the frame to carry books, etc.

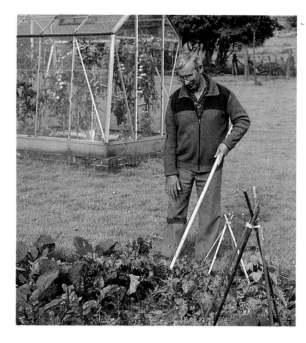

377 Advanced walking. In the later stages of treatment the patient should practise walking on carpets, out of doors, on rough ground, slopes, steps and stairs. He should open doors, reach up and down, and pick things up from the floor.

Activities of daily living

In the days following a stroke the patient may be able to do very little for himself. It is important to make the most of every achievement, helping him into a position where he can drink independently, at least wash his face, and comb his hair. The patient needs to regain a measure of independence, especially in personal care. He needs to see improvement to maintain his motivation and combat depression. The occupational therapist will design a programme to guide the patient through activities such as washing, dressing, eating, cooking and housework. Activities will be broken down into stages and realistic goals are set at each stage.

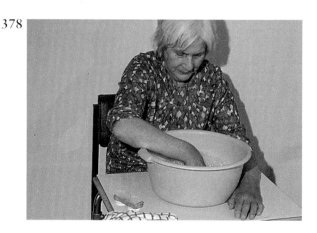

378 Washing. The patient may find it easier to wash using a bowl of water sitting at a table rather than lying in bed.

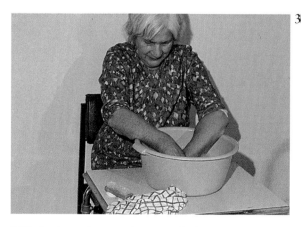

379 As the patient regains control of movement the affected hand can be safely washed in the bowl if the patient is sitting at a table. A suction nail brush is useful for the sound hand.

380 Examples of bath aids. Even in the late stages getting in and out of a bath requires a lot of effort, especially for the elderly. The occupational therapist can advise on suitable aids, such as a bath board, bath seat, non-slip mat, grab rail and shower.

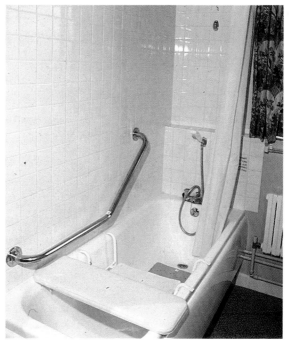

Comfortable clothes should be chosen that are not too tight, and preferably those that will stretch and have easy, accessible fastenings or, where possible, no fastenings at all. The patient should choose which clothes to wear and should be pleased with his appearance — this will help boost his morale. The patient should be sitting in a good position to dress, with weight going through both sides equally. Sitting in an armchair encourages the patient to slump back, and the back rest and chair arms get in the way. When dressing, the patient must remain relaxed. If he becomes frustrated spasticity may increase, making it even harder to dress the affected side.

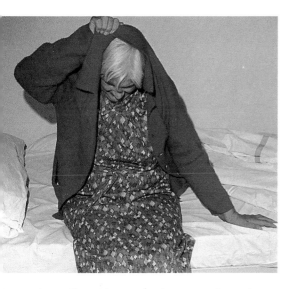

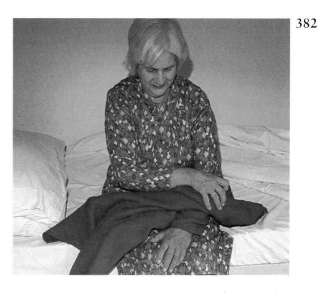

381 Taking off a cardigan, vest, dress, etc. After making sure the patient is not sitting on the garment, it can be pulled forward over the head by the sound arm, with the affected arm weight-bearing in extension. This movement should not involve much effort and avoids adverse movement of the affected side.

382 The sound arm should be taken out first, then the sleeve eased off the affected arm. Attempting to pull the affected arm out of the sleeve would involve flexion and most likely increase spasticity.

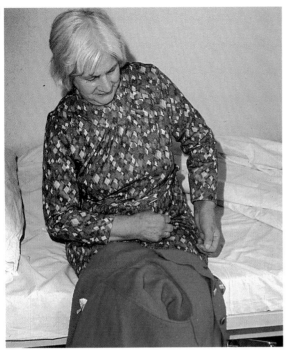

383 Putting on a sleeve. Harmful: trying to lift the affected arm is very tempting but involves flexion and visibly increases spasticity, making it almost impossible to get the hand — now a fist — into the sleeve.

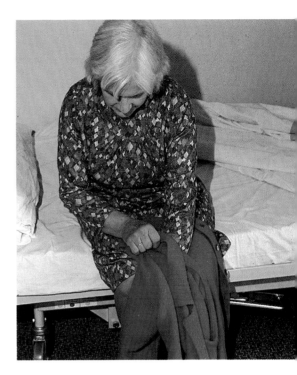

384 The cardigan should be organised so that the armhole is visible and the sleeve hanging free. The patient leans forward, sliding the arm into the sleeve using protraction of the shoulder and extension of the elbow.

It often requires less effort to put the garment over the head before putting the sound arm in, particularly garments such as jumpers and vests.

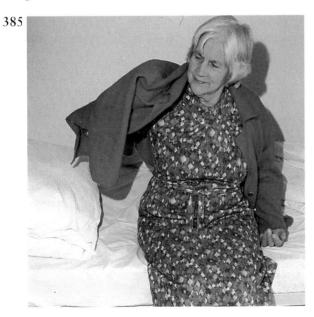

385 Putting the sound arm into a sleeve. Harmful: the patient is trying to reach up for the sleeve. This encourages retraction of both shoulders and increases spasticity, especially if the patient is not weight-bearing on the affected arm.

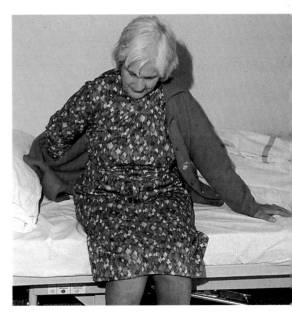

386 Reaching down for the sleeve encourages leaning forward, which avoids retraction of the affected shoulder.

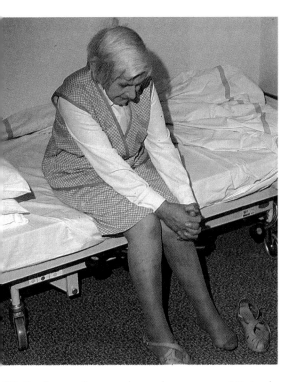

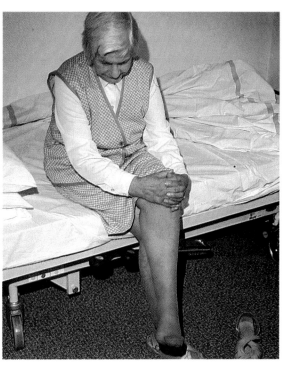

387 **Putting on shoes, socks, underpants, etc.** Minimal effort is involved if the patient can use clasped hands to cross the affected leg over the sound leg.

388 This is preferable to attempting to lift the leg on its own, which may increase spasticity.

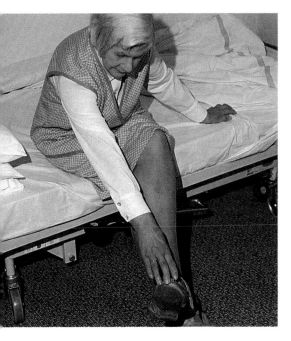

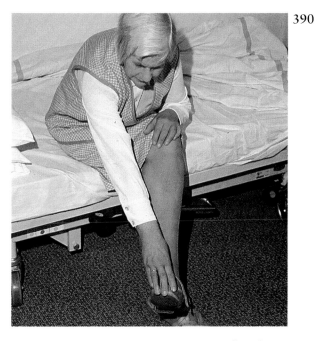

389 The patient leans forward to put the garment over the affected foot. The affected arm should be weight-bearing to counteract the adverse postural effects of increased effort.

390 If the patient has difficulty getting the affected arm into a weight-bearing position and finds it impractical during dressing, the affected hand can be placed on the knee, but should not be tucked in flexion on the patient's lap.

391

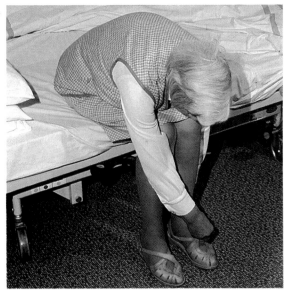

Note that after putting both legs into a garment (e.g. underpants) the patient should stand to pull the garment up. This is important to achieve independence for toileting.

391 The patient leans right forward to fasten the shoe. The affected arm should never remain tucked in the lap, but should reach down to the floor, providing trunk extension, shoulder protraction and extension of the arm. Leaning forward helps to reduce the fear of falling and leads to a better pattern of standing up.

The patient may need to have some fastenings on his clothes altered and may need to learn new techniques such as a one-handed method of tying shoelaces. If the patient has difficulties, for example because of arthritis, dressing aids may be required.

392

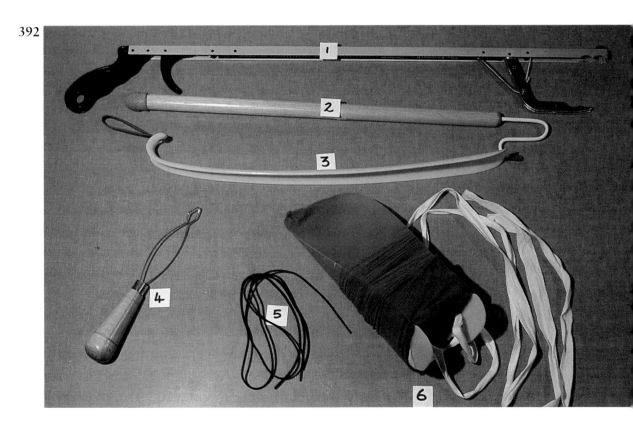

392 Examples of dressing aids. 1 Helping hand reacher, **2** Dressing stick, **3** Shoehorn, **4** Button hook, **5** Elastic shoelaces, **6** Stocking aid.

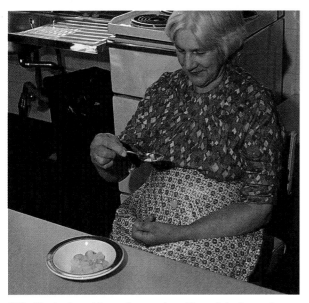

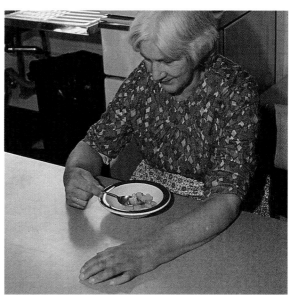

393 Typical position when eating. Harmful: the patient is leaning back with neck flexed. Food is often spilt on the long journey from plate to mouth. The arm is tucked in flexion on the patient's lap.

394 Correct position when eating. The patient is leaning forward, reducing neck flexion. Food is more likely to reach the mouth without spilling. The patient is weight-bearing through the forearm on a table of suitable height.

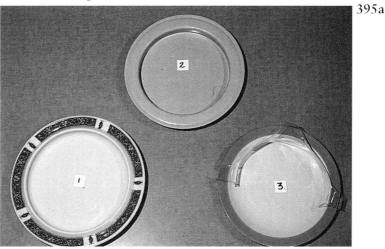

395a

395 a) Examples of eating aids. 1 and **2** Specially designed rimmed plates. **3** Plate guard.

The patient is able to push food against a lip on the plate to avoid it spilling on to the table.

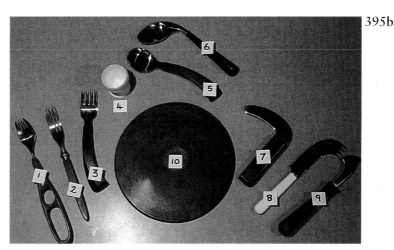

395b

395 b) 1 Fork with easy grip. **2** Fork with cutting edge. **3** Left-handed fork. **4** Suction egg cup. **5** Right-handed spoon. **6** Angled spoon. **7** Curved angled knife. **8** Knife and fork combined. **9** Angled knife. **10** Non-slip mat.

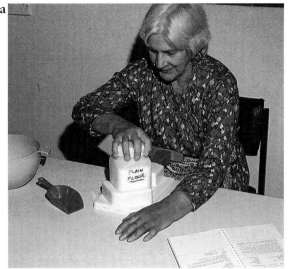

396a

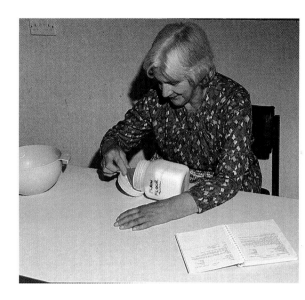

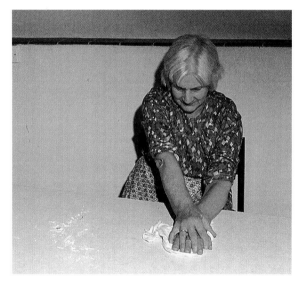

396c

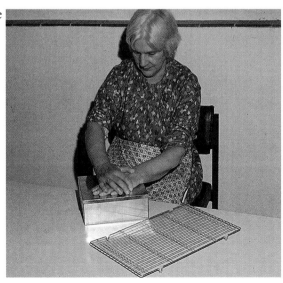

396e

396 a) **Food preparation.** If there is insufficient recovery in the affected arm the patient will find it impractical to involve it. Weight-bearing on the forearm will inhibit spasticity and the patient will achieve trunk rotation while reaching across for ingredients. A clamp holds the container still.

b) **Tipping the container** makes it easier to spoon out the ingredients.

c) **Bilateral pastry rolling** is possible, but can increase spasticity if the patient has insufficient control. The pastry rarely comes out evenly and the patient may prefer to use the sound arm only.

d) **Bilateral wiping** of the table is an excellent activity, involving weight transference, trunk extension and rotation as well as assisted arm movement.

e) The affected arm could be used in things like pressing on lids, but the patient is likely to find it impractical.

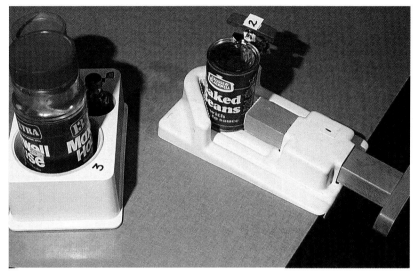

397 a) Examples of kitchen aids. 1 Clamp for holding items steady. **2** Can opener. **3** Non-spill jar and bottle opener.

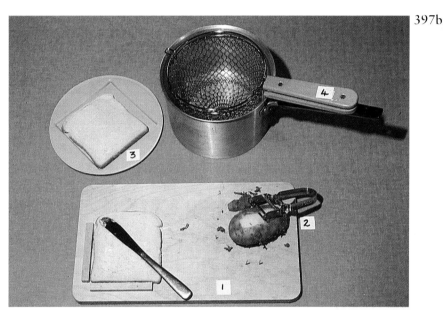

397 b) 1 Breadboard, **2** Potato peeler, **3** Bread and butter plate, **4** Cooking basket.

Many patients live alone and will have to achieve a high standard of independence if they are to cope at home. The hospital-based multidisciplinary team will need to discuss the patient's progress and make realistic recommendations. The occupational therapist should carry out home visits before discharge so that the patients can practise activities of daily living in their own home.

Adjustments in the house and living arrangements may have to be made to enable the patient to cope, for example bringing the bed downstairs to the ground floor or fitting a second bannister. Additional equipment may be needed, such as a chemical commode or chair-raising blocks. The patient will need help from the community and social services with activities like bathing, shopping and laundry.

The house may be unsuitable for the patient's residual ability and he may have to face rehousing. Support from relatives and help from the social worker will be required.

After discharge, the patient may need to attend the hospital (for physiotherapy, occupational therapy, speech therapy or day hospital) or an outpatient facility for continuing rehabilitation (see section on the stroke patient at home).

Coping with complications

Painful shoulder

This is a common complication in the hemiplegic patient. It occurs because the lack of tone in the muscles around the shoulder joint renders it unprotected and unstable. If the arm is unsupported, gravity may cause a drag on the shoulder, pulling the ball of the joint out of the socket (subluxation). Movements of the arm will be painful but subluxation can be painless.

In addition, the muscles around the shoulder joint may develop spasticity. This prevents normal movement, therefore any passive movements that forcibly oppose the spastic resistance will cause trauma and pain.

Finally, repetitive incorrect handling of the patient will result in a very painful shoulder. Care must be taken to avoid any lifting under the affected shoulder – this could cause subluxation and even dislocation.

Prevention and treatment. Correct lifting techiques must be used by everyone handling the patient. While the shoulder is painful, the patient should be encouraged not to sit and 'nurse' it. In the spastic patient, careful mobilisation of the shoulder can be carried out by the physiotherapist to relieve pain. If the shoulder joint is continuously painful, medical treatment will be required, such as ultrasound and steroid injections.

The wearing of a shoulder support can counteract gravity. It can be used to protect the shoulder as a preventive measure, and can also relieve pain if the shoulder has already been damaged.

398

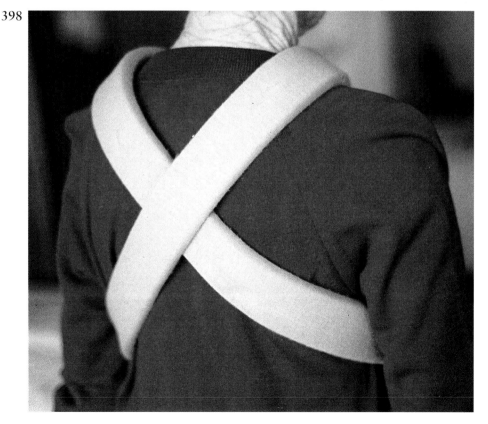

398 Correct support.
A figure of eight bandage supports the shoulder but leaves the arm free.

Oedema

A common complication of hemiplegia caused by the lack of activity in the affected arm and leg is disuse oedema. The muscle pump that normally works to prevent tissue fluid from building up in the extremities is lost. Routine use of elastic stockings aims to prevent oedema and venous thrombosis. Passive movements can be carried out by the physiotherapist. Positioning the arm in elevation on a pillow and the leg on a stool will use gravity to help reduce the swelling.

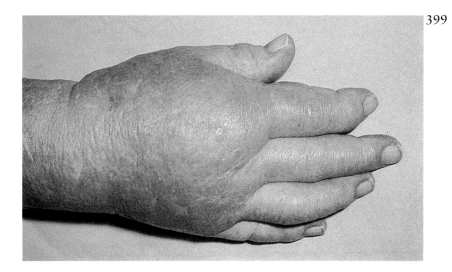

399

399 Oedema of the hand with hemiplegia. Similar oedema can occur in the lower limbs.

Gross spasticity

Some patients experience severe, stubborn spasticity in the arm and leg, particularly in the fingers and toes. It is important to obtain extension. This can be encouraged by the use of finger and toe spreaders. These should be comfortable and can also be worn in bed. The toe spreader can be worn in the patient's shoe when walking and often improves the quality of his gait.

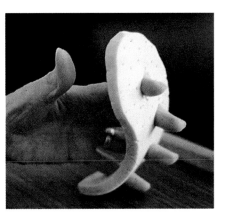

400 Finger spreader.

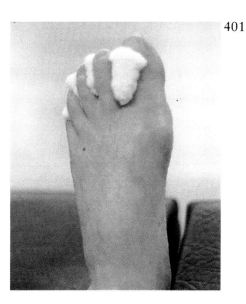

401

401 Toe spreader.

Acknowledgement
We would like to acknowledge Mrs Berta Bobath, MBE, FCSP, for her devoted work with hemiplegic patients, and whose principles we have followed in this chapter.

PERCEPTUAL PROBLEMS

Pauline Watson

Perception can be described as the understanding of sensory stimuli and the ability to relate them to past experience.

Problems of neglect, lack of recognition and disturbed spatial relationships occur more often with damage to the non-dominant side of the brain. Problems of motor control and language difficulties tend to be more common with damage to the dominant side of the brain.

With perceptual problems the patient can have a distorted view of himself, which hampers recovery of the affected side and can rob him of the desire to move. He may have a distorted view of the environment, which makes it difficult and dangerous to move around and to attempt to use objects when, for example, cooking a meal.

Treatment

The occupational therapist can assess the patient to discover the nature of the disorder. It can then be explained to the patient and his relatives. The patient may feel that he is becoming demented if he can no longer read the newspaper, feed himself or pour a cup of tea. Frequently he is in danger of being labelled as confused, lazy, or unco-operative, and then treated as such. This can adversely affect his morale and can cause him to become aggressive.

It is important to break activities down into stages, to give clear instructions, use repetition and set realistic goals.

The problems can be grouped into three sections:

- Neglect of the affected side.

- Problems of recognition and spatial relationships.

- Problems of motor planning.

Neglect of the affected side

Loss of sensation. Homonymous hemianopia and loss of sensation on the affected half of the body can both cause neglect. However, this results from loss of stimuli rather than a perceptual disorder.

402a

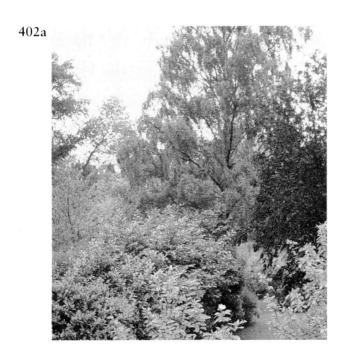
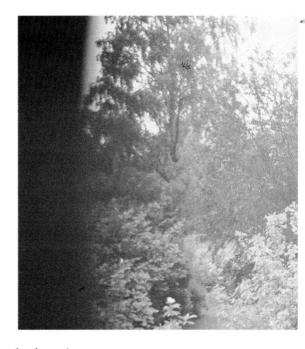

402 a) and b) **Hemianopia.** Only half of the visual field is seen by the patient.

Unilateral neglect. Sensory input from the affected side of the body and the environment may be intact, but the patient is unable to recognise the presence of anything on that side.

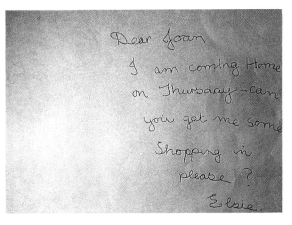

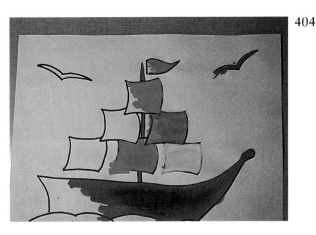

404

403 Reading and writing. The patient will read only half of each line of writing, and will write on only half the page.

404 Painting. The patient has left-sided hemiplegia. Only the right half of each section is painted correctly, failing either to meet or stop at the borders on the left.

405a

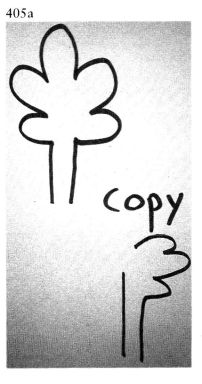

405b

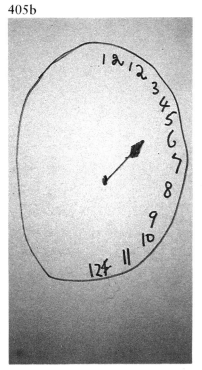

405c

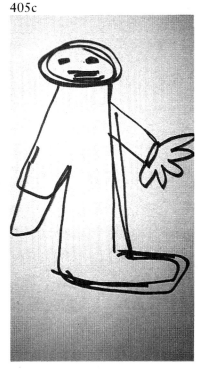

405 a) Copying a drawing. The patient will copy only the right half of a drawing.

405 b) Drawing a clock. All twelve figures may be fitted into the right side of the circle.

405 c) Perception of a person. The patient ignores the left half of the figure.

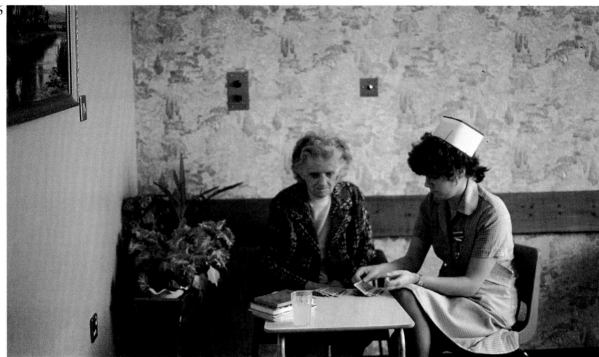

406 Position in the room. The bed and armchair can be positioned so that stimulation, in the form of familiar objects, visitors, noise, etc., comes from the affected side. Care should be taken that the patient does not become too isolated.

In treatment the patient should be encouraged to look at his affected side and assisted to wash and dress it himself. Weight-bearing and touch are important.

Food and drink should be placed on the neglected side, but the patient will need assistance in order to find them. Bilateral activities that cross into the neglected side are useful.

Right/left discrimination. The patient may lose the concept of right and left, both in relation to himself and to the environment. This can cause confusion and disorientation.

Body scheme disturbance. Body image recognition is the way we feel about our bodies, e.g. fat or thin, handsome or ugly. Body scheme refers to the way we think our body is structured — the parts that make it up, their relation to each other and their position in space. With body scheme disturbance the patient mistakes one part of his body for another, and his own body with that of someone else. Without knowing the position of his body it is difficult for him to move it from one place to another.

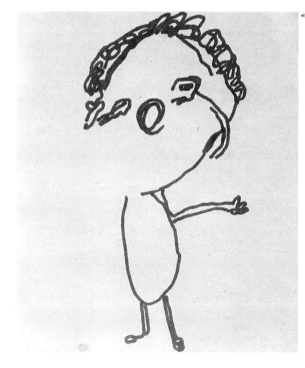

407 Missing body parts. In drawing, the patient may miss out a limb altogether. Unilateral neglect can contribute to body scheme disorder.

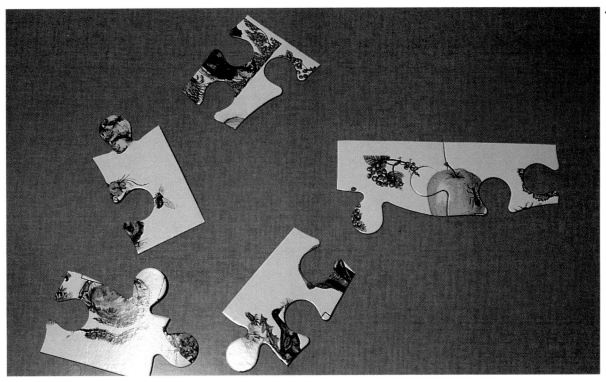

408 a) Jigsaw puzzle. The patient may be able to complete a jigsaw . . . **b)** but not if the picture is of a body. Tact and care should be exercised in conducting these tests as they may irritate and upset the patient.

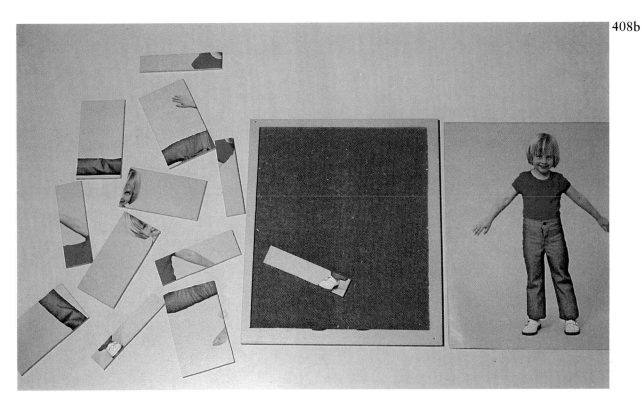

Problems of recognition and spatial relationships

Agnosia is failure to recognise the make-up of the body. Body scheme disturbances, including anosognosia, are forms of agnosia.

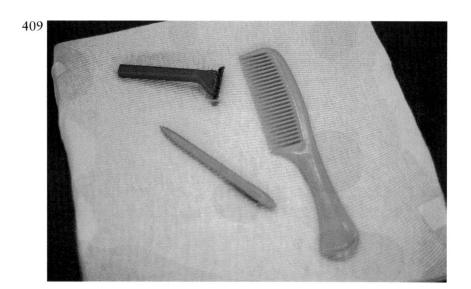

409 Visual agnosia. The patient often puts objects such as razor, comb and pen in his mouth, as a young child would when exploring an unfamiliar object. He may fail to recognise faces, photographs and colours.

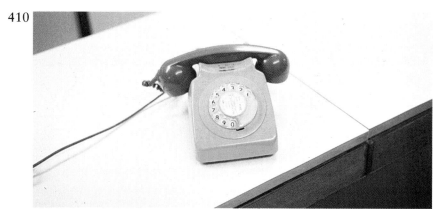

410 Auditory agnosia. The patient fails to recognise sounds such as the telephone ringing.

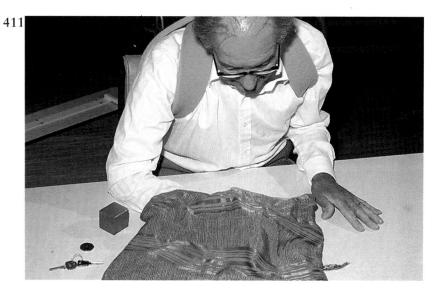

411 Astereognosis. The patient is unable to recognise an object by touch.

Anosognosia is a condition where the patient fails to recognise his disability. He may feel that his arm is missing or is not a part of his body. He will neglect to use it. The occupational therapist can help by practising activities such as body jigsaw puzzles and naming parts of the body, particularly during dressing practice.

Spatial disorders. The patient has disturbed perception of the relationship between two objects or between himself and an object. Perception of depth and distance is disturbed and the patient can lose orientation, for example, he may be unable to find his way to the toilet.

412 Visual spatial agnosia. The patient has difficulty putting two objects together, e.g. cup and saucer. He may have difficulty locating the cup to pick it up again.

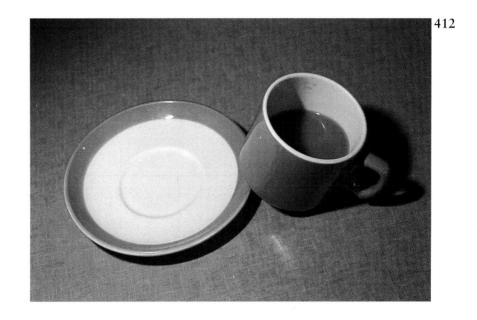

412

413 Form constancy. The patient may think that two objects of similar shape are identical, for example a comb and a pen.

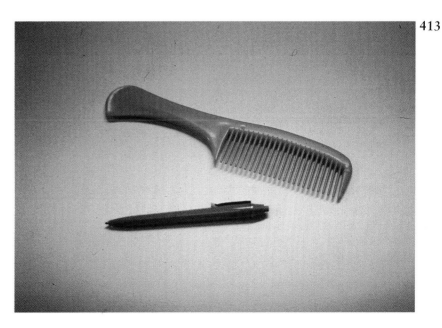

413

414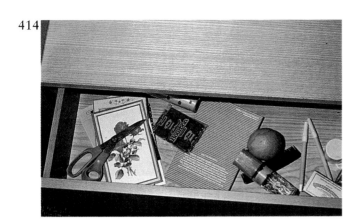

414 Figure-ground discrimination. The patient cannot distinguish foreground from background, cannot see one shape in a collection of shapes, nor find one object from a group in his drawer.

The occupational therapist can work with the patient using remedial games that concentrate on skills such as picking up objects, placing two objects together, and matching like objects.

415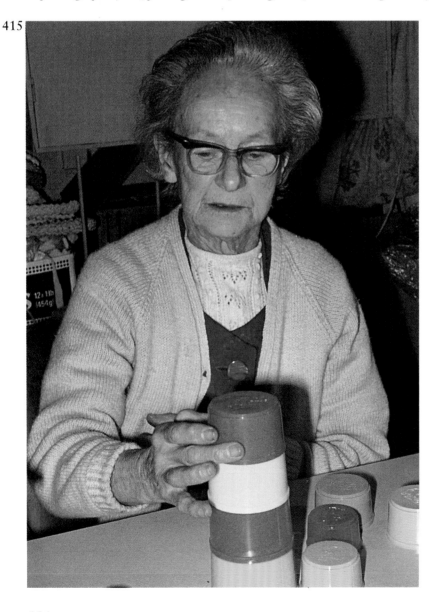

415 Remedial game. Placing objects together.

Problems of motor planning (apraxia)

The patient has lost the pattern of sequencing a movement. Even if she understands the task and has sufficient movement to perform it, she is unable to plan the required sequence to achieve the goal.

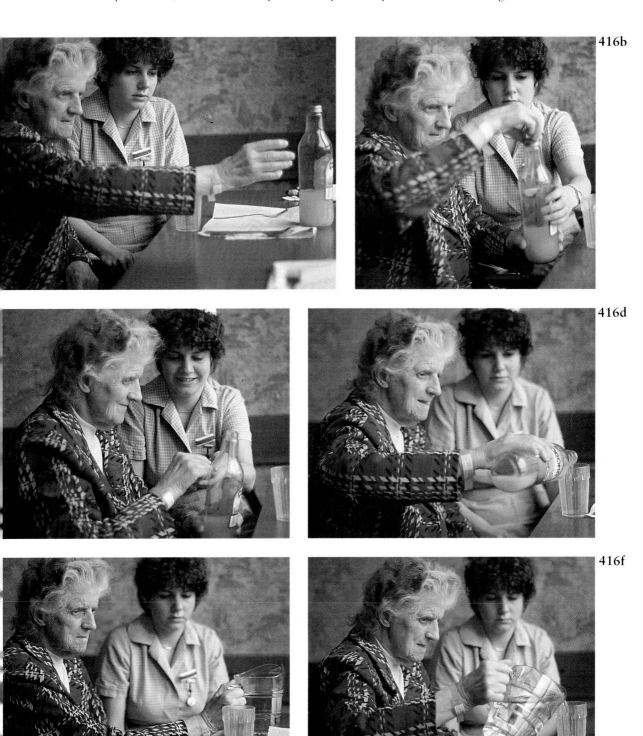

416b

416d

416f

416 a), b), c), d), e), and **f) Sequencing.** Even a simple task, such as pouring a drink from a bottle, can be too difficult.

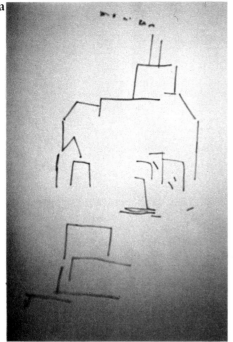

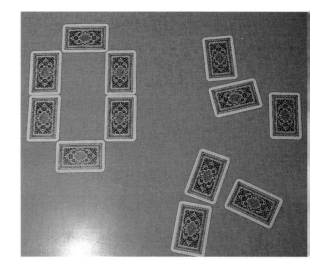

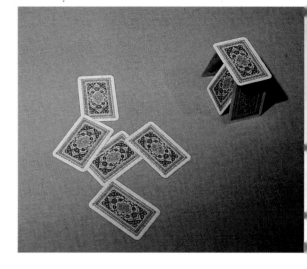

417 Constructional apraxia. a) The patient is unable to copy by drawing; **b)** to copy a two-dimensional design, or **c)** a three-dimensional design.

Some patients are able to perform familiar tasks spontaneously, but are unable to perform on command or to learn new tasks. The occupational therapist must examine each activity and break it down into stages, presenting the patient with only one step at a time.

SPEECH THERAPY

Lauri Softley

The aims of treating speech and language disturbance in the stroke patient are the restoration of an effective communication system and the readjustment of the patient and family to changes in the ways they can communicate. The aims are met by the twin processes of assessment and therapy. Assessment investigates the physical, linguistic and cognitive impairments that underly the disruption in language performance.

Dysphasia

Dysphasia is an acquired language disturbance following brain injury. The individual shows a diminished ability to interpret or use all aspects of language, i.e. speaking, writing, reading or understanding spoken language.

Assessment

Investigation of the language deficit shows the ability to retrieve words, to select and sequence the sounds of an intended word and to use the grammatical framework that encodes meaning. Identified impairments affect both expressive and receptive functions. Examples are:

Broca's dysphasia: non-fluent dysphasia (also known as expressive dysphasia or efferent motor dysphasia). There is characteristic halting output of words, with a restriction on the complexity of grammatical relationships expressed. Speech is awkward and difficult. Defects of auditory comprehension are evident on testing, and patients show impaired speech melody, dyslexia (reading difficulties) and dysgraphia (writing difficulties).

Wernicke's dysphasia: fluent dysphasia (also known as receptive dysphasia or acoustic dysphasia). Speech output is fluent with smooth easy articulation, but is disrupted by the characteristic appearance of unintended sounds, syllables or words (jargon). Auditory comprehension is markedly impaired and there is a poor awareness of errors. Appropriate use of sophisticated grammatical forms is evident, but there is a notable lack of the nouns and verbs. There is also dyslexia and dysgraphia.

Conduction dysphasia (afferent motor dysphasia). Patients have fluent, grammatically well-organised output with some errors of sound selection. Word-finding is a problem, but there is good auditory comprehension and good awareness of errors leading to typical attempts at correction. Repeating phrases or sentences is difficult for this group.

Global dysphasia. There is gross impairment of all aspects of language performance, and speech output is severely limited.

Associated non-language difficulties. There may be associated problems that require assessment:

Identification of sensory deficits, such as peripheral or cortical deafness, reduced visual acuity, or visual field defects.

Neuropsychological evaluation, such as auditory recognition and auditory memory, visual recognition, investigation of dyspraxia, attention loss, orientation and level of alertness, memory loss and reduced initiative.

Differential diagnosis of dementia. There will be typically inappropriate responses, and other features of dementia.

Communication status, such as premorbid language skills, e.g. social background, use of compensatory strategies, e.g. gesture, and reaction to loss of function, e.g. depression, anxiety.

During assessment the speech therapist will identify areas of language strength and weakness, the communication needs of the patient and his family, together with some indications of the likely prognosis. This allows decisions to be made regarding the overall aims of the therapy programme, the type of therapy needed and the most effective means of presentation. Periodic reassessment is necessary to evaluate progress and redefine therapy goals.

Formal aphasia testing investigates the understanding of spoken and written language and the expressive skills of reading and writing. Standard tests in common usage in speech therapy clinics are: the Boston Diagnostic Aphasia Examination;[7] the Minnesota Test for Differential Diagnosis of Aphasia;[8] The Porch Index of Communicative Ability,[9] and the Western Aphasia Battery.[10]

A second group of tests explores the patient's functional level of communication, i.e. how well he can use his language in everyday situations. Examples are the Functional Communication Profile;[11] and Communicative Abilities in Daily Living.[12]

Aims of treatment are:

- To promote the recovery of disrupted language processes using specific techniques.

- To enhance the communicative effectiveness of remaining/recovering language by compensatory strategies (e.g. gesture, drawing, symbol/picture selection boards, use of more sophisticated electronic communication aids).

- To stimulate functional use of the communication system available.

- To counsel relatives and staff about how to help the dysphasic patient by making changes in their own speech and language behaviour.

- To inform about self-help groups or other professional agencies who may be of value to the patient or his family during rehabilitation.

Individual treatment sessions are arranged, either on an intensive daily basis or at intervals. Therapy schedules are usually as follows:

1 Where language skills are not lost but stroke damage has made them less accessible to the patient, repeated controlled **stimulation** of these skills improves function. Language stimulation can focus on a particular receptive or expressive skill, or can emphasise the functional aspects of communication, e.g. PACE therapy (Promoting Aphasics' Communicative Effectiveness) encourages communication by any means that ends in a successful message.

2 Where language abilities are lost, undamaged brain tissue, including the right hemisphere, can be used in promoting their recovery. Therapy tasks aim at **reorganisation** of lost abilities, step by step, integrating simpler language skills into more complex and sophisticated levels of ability, e.g. melodic intonation therapy uses the preserved right hemisphere's involvement in processing melody and rhythm to stimulate expressive language in severely non-fluent dysphasic patients.

3 Where some language skills are irreversibly lost, the aim of therapy is to stimulate the development of 'cueing' or self-help behaviours. For example, a severely non-fluent dysphasic patient was given a small cut-out of the mouth position that begins the name 'Eileen'. This helped him to recall his wife's name whenever he ran his fingers over the card in his pocket.

Group treatment sessions bring the patient closer to real life. They encourage interaction and allow patients to practise the social behaviour that governs communication. In some areas there are Stroke Clubs, where information is exchanged and advice and support is available to the stroke patient and his family.

Factors affecting the recovery of speech and language skills

- The site and extent of the lesion.

- A previous history of stroke illness.

- Age.

- The time since the onset.

- The presence of associated deficits (e.g. hearing loss).

- The intellectual status of the individual.

- The level of auditory comprehension.

- The patient's personal attitude, awareness and motivation.

- The help and support available from the patient's environment.

- The general health of the patient.

Dysarthria

Dysarthria is a collective term describing motor speech disturbances following damage to those parts of the nervous system innervating the vocal mechanism. It describes a reduction in the intelligibility of spoken language and not a dysfunction of the language being expressed. Dysarthria and dysphasia may coexist in the same patient.

Assessment. Dysarthria evaluation shows the relative strength, range and accuracy of movement of the different parts of the speech apparatus. Impaired function in the mechanism of respiration, phonation, resonance and articulation causes errors of sound production, inappropriate pitch levels and changes in vocal quality. Dysphagia (swallowing difficulties) may also exist. This demands a separate detailed examination, to assess the efficiency of the three phases of the swallowing process — oral, pharyngeal and oesophageal.

Treatment. Dysarthria treatment aims to identify ways in which the patient can maximise his potential for the recovery of damaged function or compensate for any residual handicap.

Techniques. Specific exercises can be done to strengthen muscle movement or improve muscular control.

Feedback instrumentation can be used to heighten an awareness of the progress made (e.g. tape recorders, sound level meters, voice operated computer programmes).

The patient can be given a device to augment or facilitate function (e.g. an amplifier, or a palatal lift when soft palate movement is impaired — velopharyngeal incompetence). Training can be given in alternative systems to augment verbal communication (e.g. gesture, or a suitable communication aid). Finally, an important part of treatment is counselling of both patient and relatives.

Dyspraxia

Dyspraxia is an impaired ability to execute an intended movement in the absence of sensory or motor dysfunction sufficient to account for the breakdown in performance. The same muscles may be seen to function adequately during automatic activities.

Assessment aims to identify the presence of a dyspraxic difficulty, differentiating faulty movements from the inco-ordination of motor origin or the incorrect responses of a receptive dysphasia.

Ideo-motor dyspraxia is difficulty in performing purposeful limb movement (e.g. waving goodbye, shaking hands).

Ideational dyspraxia is difficulty in completing an accurate gesture demonstrating object usage.

Orofacial dyspraxia is difficulty in performing voluntary movements of speech mechanism, including respiration and phonation.

Verbal dyspraxia is difficulty with sequencing the muscle movements during intended single sound production or longer sound sequences.

Treatment consists of providing the patient with a multisensory therapy that aims at controlled production of the lost movement. Multisensory therapy involves visual, tactile and auditory input. Treatment proceeds through closely defined steps of difficulty, so that the patient has to master one step before progressing to the next. In the treatment of a dyspraxia long, demanding drilling is needed to re-establish accurate sound production. A period of auditory training is usual to improve patient awareness.

Treatment can include the introduction of alternative communication aids to augment speech during recovery.

Guidelines for helping stroke patients with speech defects

- Seek expert advice from a speech therapist.
- Check for deafness.
- Check hearing aid is functional.
- Speak clearly, using short sentences and single commands, and listen to the patient carefully.
- Encourage him to write if this is possible.
- Avoid tests and questions that may be discouraging.
- Do not bombard the patient with demands for speech.
- Develop communication by ANY means.
- Be optimistic.
- Discuss current affairs and old interests.
- Read to him to provide new topics of conversation.
- Encourage visitors and friends to reassure him of his continuing worth in social situations.
- Do not speak as if the patient were of low intelligence or a child.
- Present things to him in his visual field.

Some patients with speech defects and perceptual problems may benefit from 'cognitive' retraining. A clinical psychologist trained in stroke rehabilitation may be able to help with such cases.

Oropharyngeal rehabilitation

Stroke may disrupt the complex neuromuscular mechanisms essential for normal chewing and swallowing. Loss of the normal guarding mechanism of the upper airway and loss of the gag reflex can result in inhalation pneumonia. Facial nerve palsy causes drooling and spillage of food. Food debris and tablets may lodge in a flaccid buccal pouch.

Ill-fitting dentures, drooping of the jaw and inability to close the mouth result in swallowing difficulties. Dental advice should be sought in cases of ill-fitting dentures resulting from gum shrinkage. If there is dryness of the mouth then dehydration should be corrected. An unstable lower denture and overspill of food into the buccal sulcus is caused by loss of function of the cheek on one side. A thickened denture base may compensate. Correct use of a palatal training appliance will reduce drooling and, to some extent, dysphagia.

Important aspects of oropharyngeal rehabilitation are:

- Attention to oral hygiene.
- Avoid dryness of mouth.
- Advise patients and relatives on correct food intake.
- Assessment of swallowing mechanism, including radiographic investigation.
- Train nurses and relatives to teach patients how to swallow.
- Correct use of drinking cups, beakers, drinking straws and other aids.

The safe-swallowing technique is used in patients with normal cough reflex:

1 Sit the patient upright.

2 A small quantity of food is placed in the mouth.

3 The patient feels the food in his mouth.

4 The patient breathes in and holds his breath.

5 While holding his breath, the patient swallows.

6 He breathes out.

7 He clears his throat.

8 Finally, he swallows, without food, to clear the oral and pharyngeal area.

9 Instruction is given throughout the swallowing process.

418

418 Speech areas in the cerebral cortex.

419 Formal assessment of **dysphasia** using the Boston Test for the Differential Diagnosis of Aphasia.

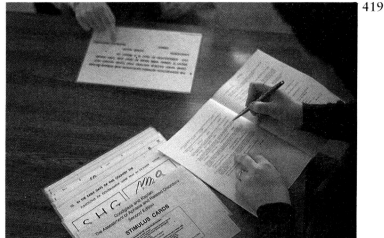

420 Material for auditory comprehension work.

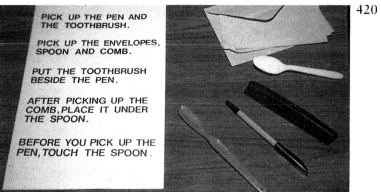

PICK UP THE PEN AND THE TOOTHBRUSH.

PICK UP THE ENVELOPES, SPOON AND COMB.

PUT THE TOOTHBRUSH BESIDE THE PEN.

AFTER PICKING UP THE COMB, PLACE IT UNDER THE SPOON.

BEFORE YOU PICK UP THE PEN, TOUCH THE SPOON.

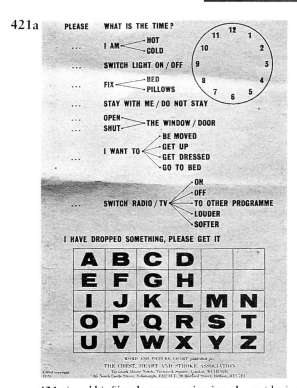

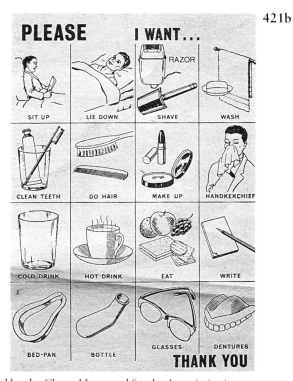

421 a) and **b)** **Simple communication charts** (devised by the Chest, Heart and Stroke Association).

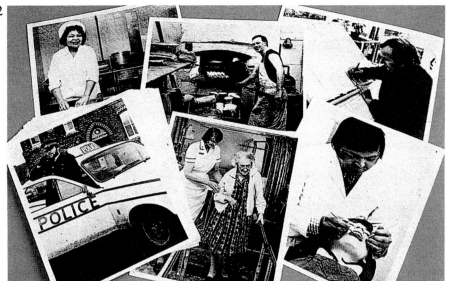

422 Conversation material — occupations.

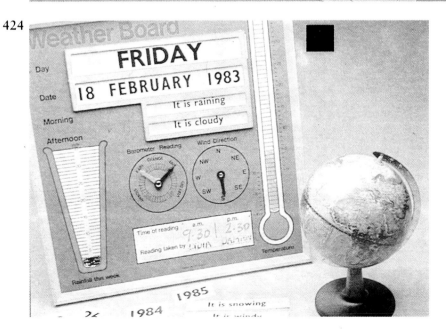

423 Conversation material — photo library.

424 Reality orientation — weather board.

425 Assessment of dysgraphic patient.

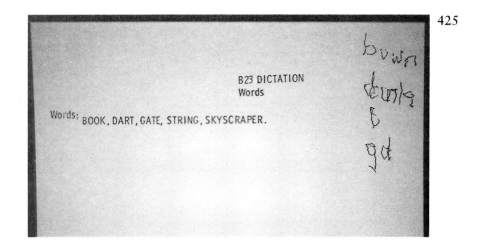

426 Simple electronic communication aid.

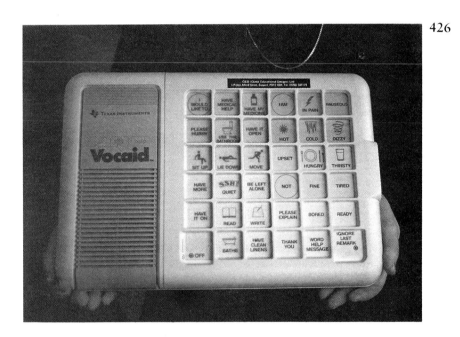

427 Material for sorting tasks with anomic patients.

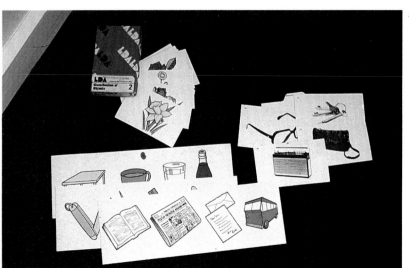

428

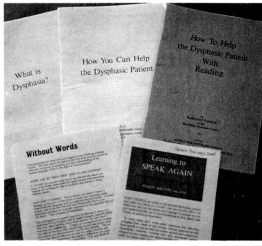

428 Material for functional reading skills.

429 Literature for family and staff.

430

430 Self-help group for dysphasic adults. Patients and relatives can be put in touch with their local branches.

431 a) Palatal lift for velopharyngeal incompetence.

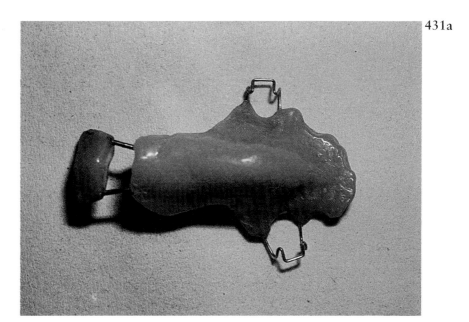

431 b) The palatal lift in position.

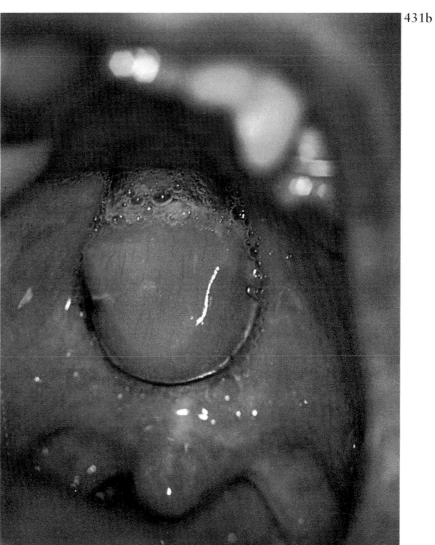

432

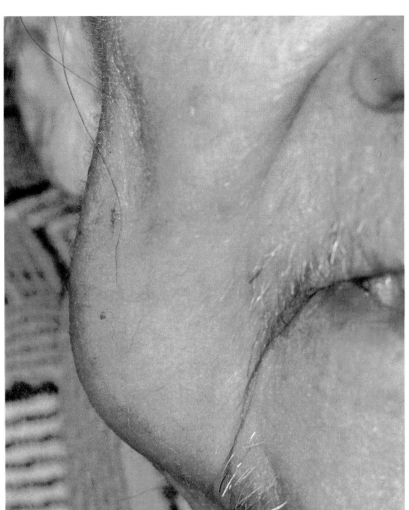

432 Buccal sulcus, caused by weakness of the cheek muscles.

433

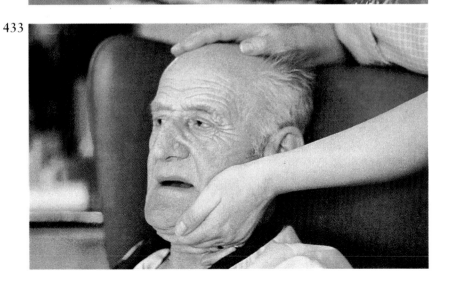

433 Therapist aiding the patient's head position and stimulating swallow.

434 A nurse assisting the patient's head position and supporting the jaw, thus assisting swallowing.

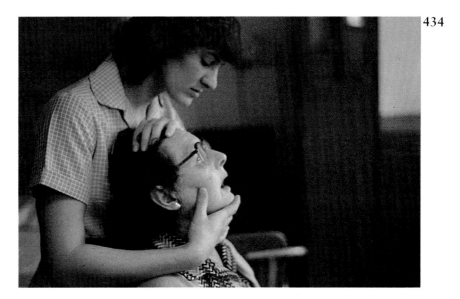

434

435 Assisting drinking by gripping the jaw to open and close the patient's mouth.

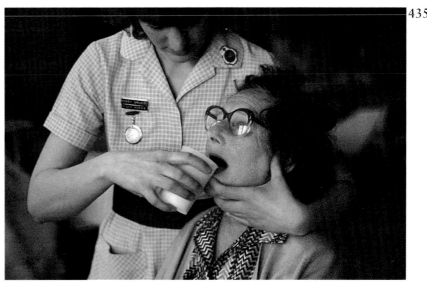

435

436 Proprioceptive neuromuscular facilitation. Some stroke patients develop oral hypersensitivity — chewing, drinking, etc., cause discomfort. Repetitive desensitisation will reduce the oral discomfort.

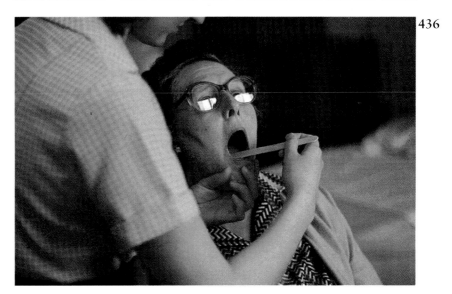

436

437

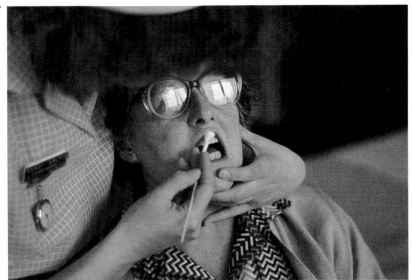

437 Gentle rubbing of the alveolar ridge for desensitisation. Such methods may be required before normal feeding.

438

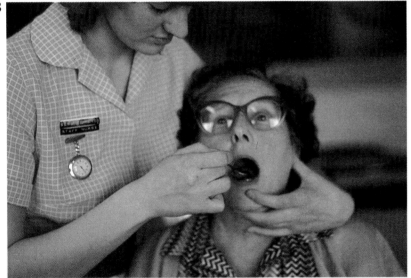

438 Jaw grip that opens the patient's mouth for feeding with a spoon.

439

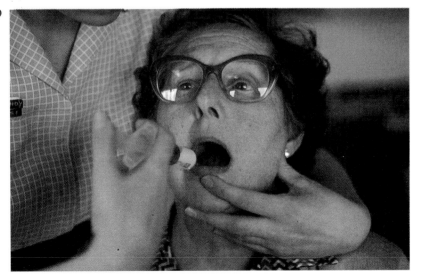

439 A syringe being used to place a small quantity of milk in the inner lip, followed by facilitated swallow.

440 Flexi-straw to help in
swallowing liquids.

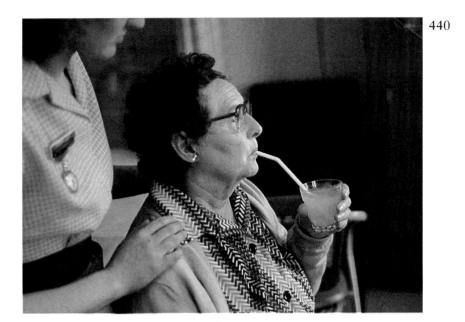

**441 Exercising the oral and
buccal muscles** by blowing soap
bubbles.

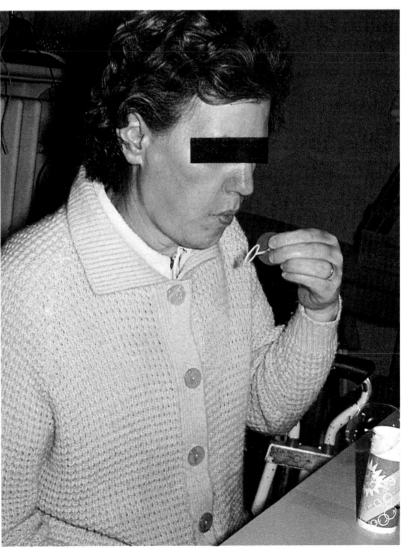

THE ROLE OF THE SOCIAL WORKER IN STROKE REHABILITATION

Sheana Bennett and Fay Killingworth

The social worker is an important member of the multi-disciplinary team (consisting of doctors, nurses, physiotherapists, occupational and speech therapists) working towards the rehabilitation of stroke patients. Ideally, social workers should be attached directly to a stroke rehabilitation ward and work with the patients and family during the period of hospitalisation as well as, most importantly, following discharge. The social worker needs to make early contact with both patient and relatives. The family and friends of the patient need a lot of help in understanding the situation and in tolerating the uncertainty about the prognosis. At this stage the social worker will be involved in the following areas:

- Providing emotional support to the patient and family, particularly in helping them to understand the implications of the illness.

- Providing a full social work report to the multi-disciplinary team with information gained from family, friends, outside agencies and domiciliary services.

- Focusing on the needs of the patient and helping him to come to terms with his condition.

- Providing practical help and advice to the patient and family, e.g. advice regarding benefits, transport for families, liaison with domiciliary services or residential establishments to notify them of the patient's current condition.

During the period of rehabilitation, a social worker may become less involved, but contributes to the work of the team in the following areas:

- Contact with the patient and also meetings with the partner and family, or whoever is closest to the patient. If there is no-one to care for the patient and help in his rehabilitation and plans for discharge then the social worker's role may become more significant regarding the overall welfare, safety and future plans for the patient.

  This is an important time in which a relationship of trust can be built up with the patient and his family. The partners of stroke victims may experience great difficulty in accepting the physical and emotional changes in someone they have known and loved. Care and understanding is required to help them to make these adjustments. The counselling skills of the social worker are important at this time.

- Practical advice and liaison with other agencies, for example in the area of housing, ground floor accommodation, warden controlled accommodation, local authority Part 3 accommodation, or private rest home or nursing home care may be required. This may necessitate meetings with housing officials, etc., and written reports to illustrate and support the patient's needs.

- Provide information and guidance regarding financial help, e.g. Supplementary Benefit, Invalidity Benefit and Non-contributory Invalidity Benefit, Attendance Allowance, Mobility Allowance, Invalid Care Allowance, Statutory Sick Pay/Sickness Benefit, Rate Rebate, or Housing Benefit.

- Advice and guidance regarding domiciliary services, e.g. home help, family aide, meals-on-wheels, night sitters, private nursing care in the home.

- Discussion, as appropriate, with the patient and his family with regard to the types of residential care available if return home is not possible. These options would need to be discussed at length, considering the practical, financial and emotional factors involved in such a decision. Visits to the various establishments would need to be made, in conjunction with the occupational therapist.

- Consideration should be given by social workers to the setting up of a group for stroke patients and a support group for the carers.

- Participation in home assessment visits in conjunction with the occupational therapist and possibly other team members.

- Participation in multidisciplinary case conferences.

Discharge and follow-up

When the time comes for the patient to go home, the social worker's role is to co-ordinate follow-up by inter-relating the various types of help available. During the weeks following discharge, the social worker must monitor the patient's progress, and may be involved in the following areas:

- Providing emotional support and counselling to the partner and family.

- Ensuring financial arrangements and benefits are progressing satisfactorily.

- Providing further support with regard to accommodation or home adaptation problems that may not have been resolved; if great difficulties arise then the option of residential care may need to be looked at again.

- Informing the patient and family of resources such as day centres for the physically handi-capped, or stroke clubs if available, and arranging attendance if necessary.

- Liaison with the Community Social Services Department.

In conclusion, the social worker has a central role to play in the care, rehabilitation and discharge of the stroke patient and in the support of his family at such a traumatic time in their lives. Imagination and creative skills are a great advantage when dealing with this particular group of patients as communication with them is often limited and difficult.

STROKE PATIENTS AT HOME

Some patients with TIAs and minor strokes can be managed at home. Disabled patients who need continuing care may be able to live at home, too, but require help and support. Patients who have recently been discharged from hospital will first have undergone a home assessment visit. These visits are conducted by the occupational therapist with support from the social worker. The patient is taken home and, preferably in the presence of the family, an assessment is made of his ability to look after himself. Also, details of accommodation are noted, as various aids and adaptations may be required, such as support rails in the bathroom and along the stairs, an emergency bell in the bathroom, an outward-opening toilet door, raised toilet seat, raised bed, specially adapted bath aids so that the patient can get in and out easily and wash himself while sitting on a small seat, and special implements, such as crockery and cutlery, e.g. long-handled brush, combined knife and fork with serrated edge, non-slip table mats, one-handed tin opener, and bed- and chair-raising blocks, wheelchair ramps, etc. Most of these have already been described in the chapter on 'Rehabilitation'.

Aids for stroke patients are available from specialist commercial companies and details can be found in their catalogues. The various Aids Centres throughout Britain give valuable help and advice on aids and adaptations for continuing re-habilitation at home and independent living. In this respect The Chest, Heart and Stroke Association has some excellent publications for both patient and family, notably *Stroke — a handbook for the patient's family* by Graham Mully,[13] *Understanding stroke illness* by Bernard Isaacs,[14] and *Home care for the stroke patient — in the early days* by Pamela Grasty.[15]

A stroke patient living independently in the community may need help from the following agencies:

- Friends and relatives.

- Family doctor.

- Social worker.

- District or private nurse.

- Domiciliary physiotherapist and occupational therapists.

- Bathing assistant.

- Voluntary organisations.

- Disablement Officer.

- Health visitor.

- Home help.

- Age Concern.

Many patients living at home continue to receive further rehabilitation at a specialist unit. This arrangement varies from place to place and can involve any one of the following: stroke rehabilitation unit (but very few available); geriatric day hospital; neurological rehabilitation unit; department of rehabilitative medicine; young chronic sick unit; day centres and social and/or luncheon clubs; stroke clubs; or industrial rehabilitation unit.

The aim of domiciliary rehabilitation is to encourage the patient to gain and maintain as much independence as possible. Help from a supportive spouse or relative is of vital importance in helping to achieve this aim.

Some helpful aids at home

- A long-handled shoe horn.
- Clothes with Velcro fastenings at the front.
- Elastic rather than cord pyjamas.
- Non-slip mats in baths and bathrails.
- Electric razors.
- Toilet frames and raised toilet seat.
- Utensils with thick handles.
- Plates with suction pads.
- Comfortable shoes.

- Furniture should be arranged in such a way that the patient can lean on it for support when getting about the house.
- Bannisters on both sides of stairs.
- Communication aid if speech is poor (simple notebook and pen!).
- Easily accessible telephone, commode and light switch.
- Adapting the kitchen for easy management.

Problems at home

The patient may experience several problems at home. The common ones are falls, urinary incontinence, constipation, pressure sores, stiffness, depression, loss or lack of motivation, poor drug compliance, malnutrition, social and emotional isolation, and financial problems.

Even a severely disabled stroke patient can lead an independent existence, but he will require physical and emotional support. The role of the family and community at large is of vital importance. Voluntary agencies and charitable organisations have an important part to play and their help should be sought at an early stage.

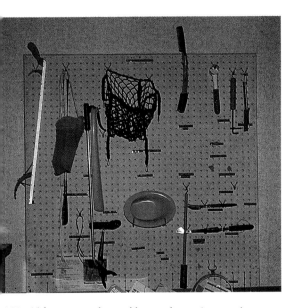

442 Aids commonly used by stroke patients at home.

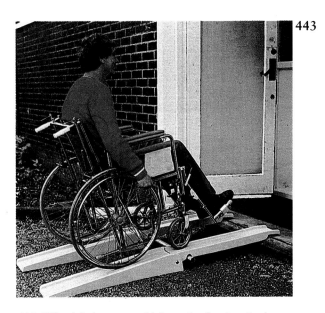

443 Wheelchair ramp, which can be fitted to the front door.

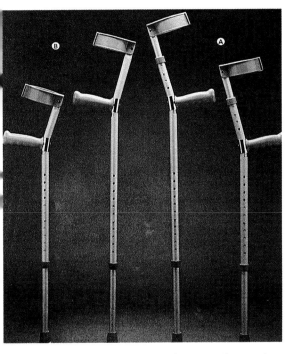

444 Adjustable elbow crutches. These crutches can be used in elderly stroke patients who suffer from arthritis. **A**) Double adjustable elbow crutch, and **B**) single adjustable elbow crutch.

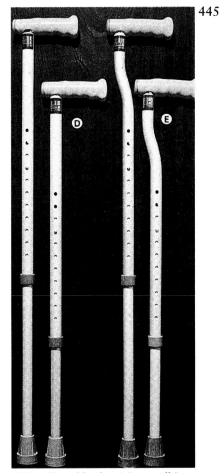

445 Adjustable aluminium walking sticks. D) Straight and **E**) swan neck.

446

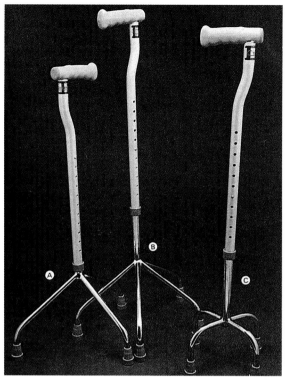

446 Tripod and tetrapod walking aids. **A)** Tripod,
B) and **C)** tetrapod.

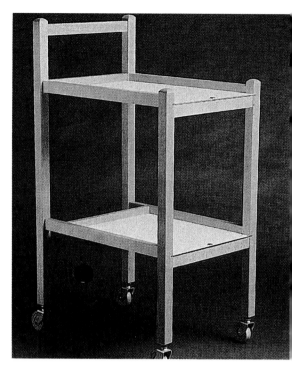

447 Trolley — especially useful for elderly patients
who are house-bound.

448

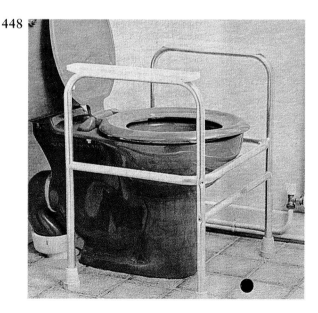

448 Toilet frame, which can be fitted around a
standard WC.

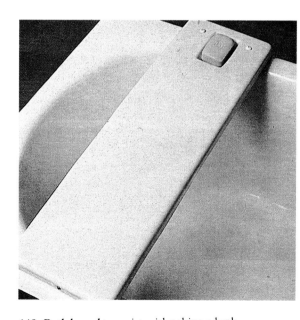

449 Bath board to assist with taking a bath.

450 Shower seat and hand rail for patients who have difficulty in getting up from a sitting position.

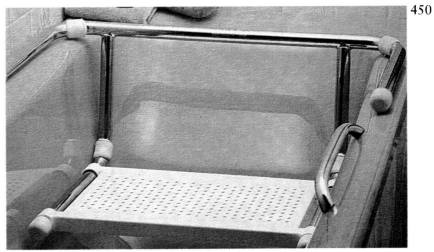

451 Adjustable bath rail to assist in getting in and out of the bath.

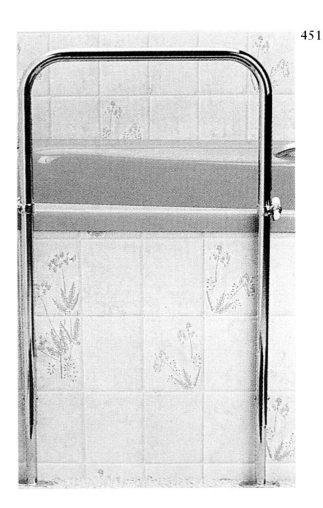

452

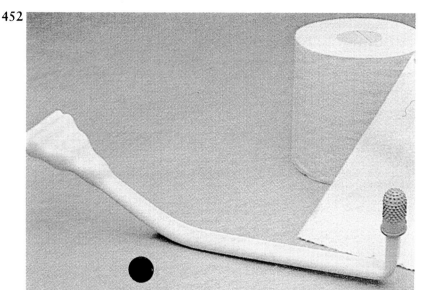

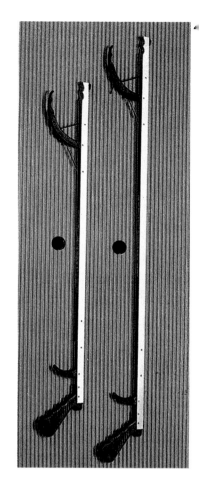

454

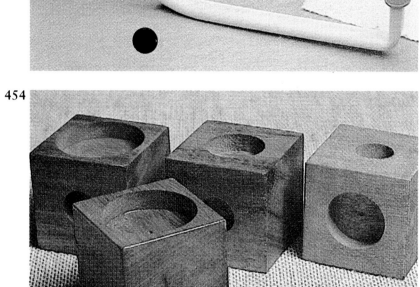

455

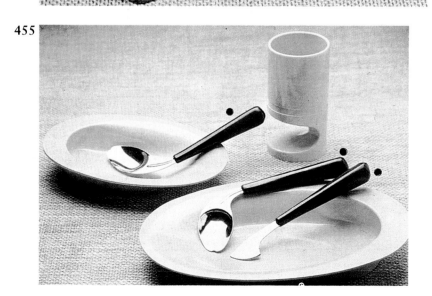

452 Bottom wiper for patients who are unable to reach with their hand.

453 Lightweight hand reachers with plastic jaws.

454 Raising blocks for beds and chairs.

455 Specially designed tableware for patients with hemiplegia.

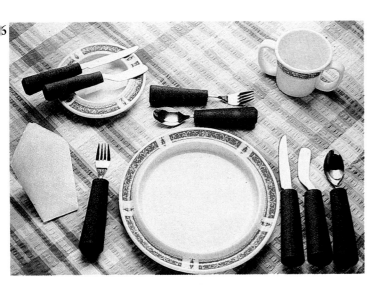

456 **Lightweight cutlery** with easy grip handles.

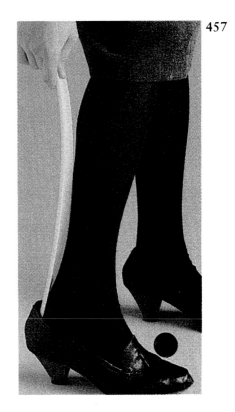

457 Long-handled shoe horn.

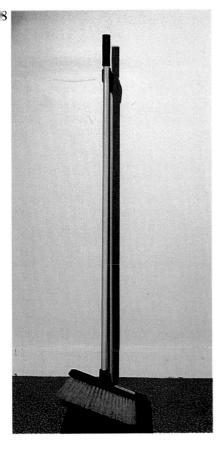

458 **Long-handled dust-pan and brush.**

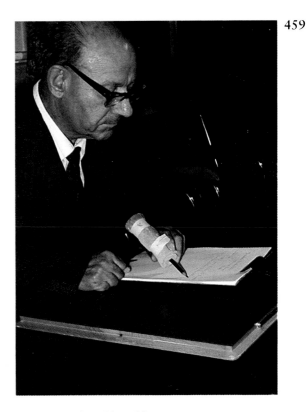

459 A simple writing aid.

460a

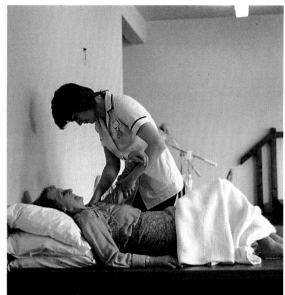

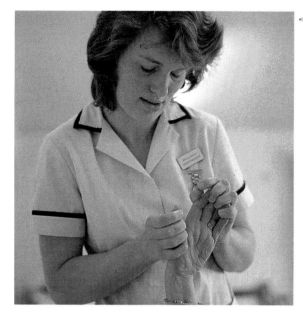

460c

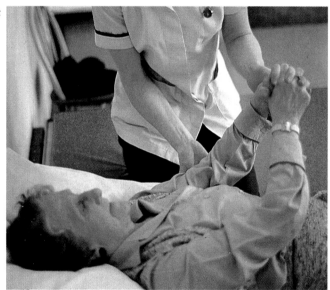

Continuing rehabilitation can be provided on an outpatient basis. **Geriatric day hospitals** are of great value in this respect.

460 a), b), c), d) and e) Physiotherapy. These pictures show various stages of maintenance physiotherapy. Here, the stroke patients attend for a course of rehabilitation at the local geriatric day hospital.

460d

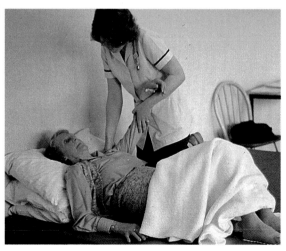

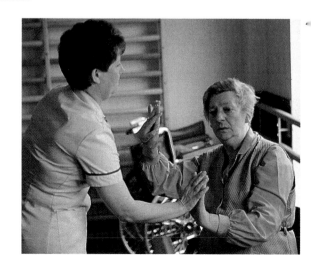

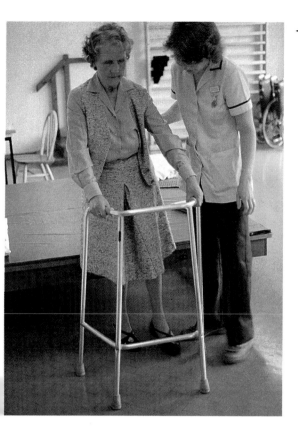

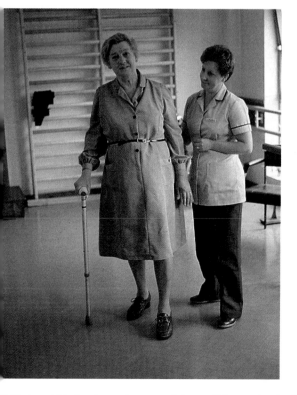

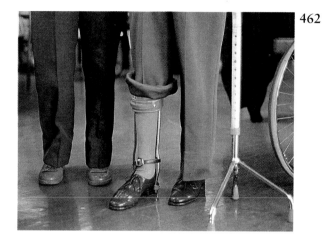

462 In some stroke patients the physiotherapist may have to resort to using splints as an aid to walking. Modern techniques of rehabilitation result in fewer patients having to use mechanical aids.

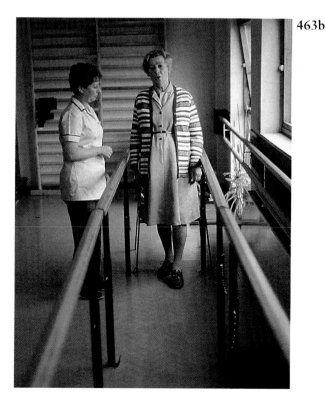

◀ **461 Stroke patient** being trained to walk with a frame.

463 a) and b) **Stroke patient practising walking** at the day hospital. Once- or twice-weekly attendances at the day hospital can enable some stroke patients to continue to manage independently at home.

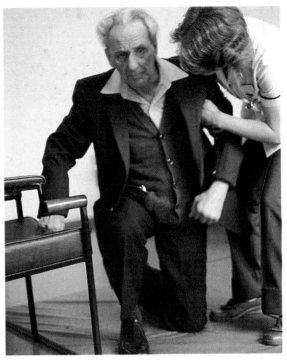

464 Stroke patient with left hemiplegia being taught to get up from the floor. Elderly stroke patients living alone are at risk from falling and may be unable to get up without assistance.

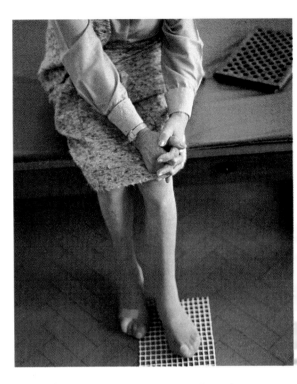

465 Non-slip mat being used to give a hemiplegic patient confidence and stability whilst standing up from a bed.

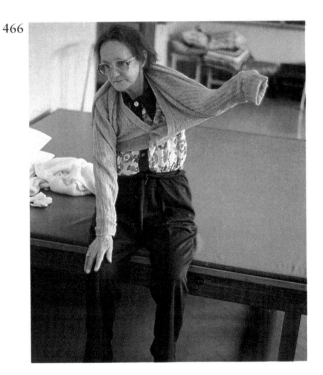

466 Stroke patient receiving dressing practice in the physiotherapy department. She attends regular 'stroke classes', along with other patients.

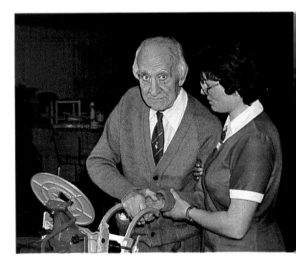

467 Patient receiving specialist therapy in handling a small printing press in the occupational therapy department.

468 Group activities. Patient and staff participation is an essential component of stroke rehabilitation.

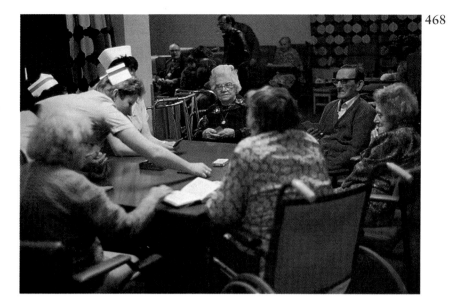

468

469 Diversional therapy in progress.

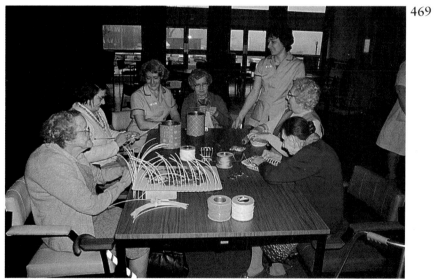

469

470 Specially adapted kitchen for patients to practise in before any changes are made in their own homes.

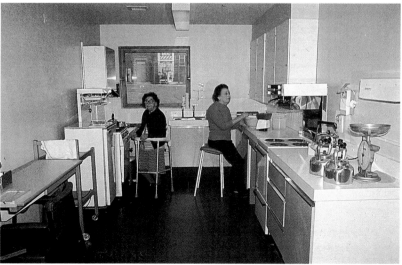

470

PREVENTION OF STROKES

There are four main areas of stroke prevention:

- Preventing atherosclerosis.
- Treatment of hypertension.
- Treatment of transient ischaemic attacks.
- Treating known aetiological factors.

Preventing atherosclerosis

Atherosclerosis is known to be associated with:

- Stress.
- Hypertension.
- Diabetes mellitus.
- Advancing age.
- A diet rich in lipid and cholesterol and low in fibre.
- Smoking.

Altering life-style and dietary habits may, to some extent, slow down the development of atheroma. Diseases that are a known risk factor for atherosclerosis need to be diagnosed and treated adequately. Good control of diabetes reduces the incidence of stroke. Smoking is harmful and patients who are predisposed to hypertension, coronary artery disease, atheroma and bronchitis must either reduce or stop smoking. Vasodilator drugs will not dilate blood vessels that have become rigid with atheroma and their benefits in treating the results of atherosclerosis are dubious. There is no convincing evidence that these drugs are beneficial in cerebral arteriosclerosis, however naftidrofuryl has been used in stroke patients with some success, particularly when given as an adjunct to rehabilitation.

Treatment of hypertension

The WHO definitions of hypertension in patients under 65 years of age are:

Normotension — less than 140/90 mm Hg.

Borderline hypertension — 140/90 to 160/95 mm Hg.

Hypertension — 160/95 mm Hg and above.

Systolic hypertension — systolic pressure greater than 160 mm Hg with diastolic pressure less than 95 mm Hg.

Diastolic hypertension — *mild* 90 to 104 mm Hg; *moderate* 105 to 120 mm Hg; *severe* greater than 120 mm Hg.

Sustained high blood pressure predisposes patients to strokes, especially cerebral haemorrhage and cerebral infarction. Hypertensives are 4 to 7 times more likely to develop strokes as normotensives. Adequate treatment of hypertension reduces the incidence of stroke. Recent research has shown that this benefit can also be obtained in elderly patients.

Most cases of hypertension are of primary type: treatable causes are found in only a minority of patients. However, all cases of hypertension require a thorough medical assessment before starting treatment.

The Medical Research Council trial of drug treatment in mild hypertension began in 1977.[2] It was a simple blind study of 17,354 patients over the age of 35 years. Subjects were randomly allocated to one of four treatment groups: bendrofluazide and identical placebo tablets, propranolol and identical placebo tablets. The trial lasted 5½ years and the results revealed that the stroke rate was reduced on active treatment. There were 60 strokes in the treated group and 109 in the placebo group, giving rates of 1.4 and 2.6 per 1,000 patient years. The stroke rate was reduced in both smokers and non-smokers taking bendrofluazide, but only in non-smokers taking propranolol. Furthermore, when hypertensives stopped smoking, the benefit was most significant. The stroke and coronary event rates were roughly halved. However, the benefits of the treatment were, to some extent, limited, as many of the patients experienced adverse drug effects.

The Veterans Administration Co-operative Study Group on Antihypertensive Agents examined the effects of treatment on morbidity in hypertension.[16] Five hundred and fifty male patients with diastolic blood pressures between 90 and 129 mm Hg were included in the trial. Eighty-one patients were over 60 years of age. The results showed that compared to placebo, active treatment was approximately 50% successful in reducing major complications, including strokes. Other studies have established the fact that good control of moderate and severe hypertension reduces the incidence of cerebral infarction and cerebral haemorrhage.

Hypertension in the elderly and its treatment have for many years been controversial. The difficulty has been in establishing the upper limits of normal blood pressure in the elderly and clarifying the indications for treatment. Indeed, many authorities maintain that postural hypotension is more dangerous in an elderly person than mild or moderate hypertension. The balance between benefit and harm is very easy to upset in the elderly, as adverse effects of therapy are common and may result in serious complications.

The European Working Party on High Blood Pressure in the Elderly (EWPHE) has attempted to answer some of the questions.[3] Their trial started in 1972. Eight hundred and forty patients with an average age of 72 years and average blood pressure of 183/101 mm Hg were included in the study. It was a multicentre, double-blind, between-patient comparison of a thiazide plus triamterene and matching placebo. The results showed that treatment had no effect on overall mortality, but cardiovascular mortality was reduced by 27%. Cerebrovascular mortality did not show any significant change but non-fatal cerebrovascular events were reduced by approximately 50%. A significant number of patients experienced adverse drug effects, particularly hypokalaemia and hyperglycaemia. However, this study has given strength to the argument that favours treating hypertension in old age. There has been some doubt as to whether one can accurately measure blood pressure in the elderly. Because of atheroma, the compliance of large blood vessels is reduced: this may give rise to 'pseudo-hypertension'. In such cases the need for therapy should be appraised by thorough assessment of cardiovascular system and renal function.

In conclusion, it may be said that in selected elderly patients, treatment of hypertension is beneficial, including the reduction of incidence of stroke and cardiovascular complications. There are a number of important considerations that need to be borne in mind before initiating antihypertensive therapy in an elderly patient:

- Quality of life.
- Mental state (?dementia).
- Co-existing disabilities.
- Drug compliance.

Antihypertensive therapy should also be considered for those patients who have already suffered a stroke, as long-term treatment does improve life expectancy.

Treatment of transient ischaemic attacks

Up to 40% of patients with TIAs have a significant risk of developing a major stroke within 2 years of the onset of TIAs. Factors contributing to the development of TIAs should be identified and

> ### Guidelines for the treatment of hypertension in the elderly
>
> 1 Carry out a full geriatric assessment.
>
> 2 Take several readings before diagnosing 'hypertension'.
>
> 3 Treat systolic blood pressure in excess of 180 mm Hg and diastolic pressure in excess of 110 mm Hg.
>
> 4 Reduce blood pressure slowly.
>
> 5 Be aware of drug interactions.
>
> 6 Treat those over 80 years of age only if there are complications, e.g. left ventricular failure or renal failure.
>
> 7 Check for postural hypotension.
>
> 8 Check drug compliance.
>
> 9 Advise the patient to stop or reduce smoking.
>
> 10 Keep an eye on plasma electrolytes and glucose.

treated, e.g. hypertension, anaemia, polycythaemia, mitral stenosis, and cardiac failure. Patients with severe atheromatous stenosis of the internal carotid artery (with or without a bruit or ulcer) and subclavian steal syndrome should be considered for surgery.

In patients where TIAs are caused by microemboli from a known source, e.g. mitral stenosis, then long-term anticoagulants should be considered. Anticoagulants are also used in patients where surgery is not contemplated and who are normotensive. Patients with frequent and disabling vertebrobasilar TIAs may also derive benefit from anticoagulant treatment. However, in elderly patients the usefulness of anticoagulants remains in doubt.

In patients where anticoagulants are contraindicated and surgery is not possible, then antiplatelet drugs should be considered. Aspirin reduces platelet stickiness and trials have shown that when given in small doses, especially to men under 55 years of age, it is effective in reducing the incidence of TIAs and transient amaurotic attacks. It may be given in doses of 75 mg once daily.

Dipyridamole reduces platelet stickiness and also causes vasodilatation. It is effective in reducing emboli from prosthetic cardiac valves and in-vitro tests have shown that, in combination with aspirin, it may be of benefit in TIAs.

Sulphinpyrazone prolongs platelet survival in vitro. There have been reports of its success in TIAs but a trial showed that when compared with aspirin it had no beneficial effects.

Treating known aetiological factors

(See also chapters on pathology, page 8, and risk factors, page 7.)

There is increased incidence of strokes in some conditions that promote atheroma, hyperviscosity, haemorrhage and thrombosis. For many of these conditions, adequate management is available. Examples are diabetes mellitus, temporal arteritis, sickle cell disease, thrombocythaemia, bacterial endocarditis, mitral stenosis and left atrial myxoma.

GLOSSARY OF TERMS

Agnosia — Failure to recognise familiar and known objects that have been perceived by the senses, e.g. touch, sight.

Agraphia — Inability to express thoughts in writing.

Alexia (dyslexia) — Difficulty in reading. Also called 'word blindness'.

Amaurosis fugax — Transient blindness in one eye.

Anomia — Inability to name familiar names and objects.

Anosmia — Inability to identify smells and odours.

Anosognosia — A perceptual problem in which the patient is unable to recognise his paralysis.

Aphasia (dysphasia) — Inability to express thoughts by speech or writing with inability to understand spoken or written language.

Apraxia (dyspraxia) — Inability to perform purposeful movements in the presence of normal motor power, sensations and co-ordination.

Astereognosis — Difficulty in recognising objects when handling and feeling them with eyes closed.

Asynergia — Defective muscle co-ordination during voluntary movements.

Ataxia — Lack of power of co-ordination during voluntary muscular motion.

Atheroma (atherosclerosis, arteriosclerosis) — Lipid deposits in the intima of large and medium-sized arteries. There is associated fibrosis and calcification. In severe cases there is progressive narrowing of the arterial lumen and thrombosis.

Athetosis — Involuntary, slow, coarse writhing movements usually in hands and arms.

Bulbar palsy — Lower motor neurone lesion of the cranial nerves 9, 10 and 12.

Cerebrovascular accident (CVA) — Damage to the brain tissue caused by a sudden reduction of the blood supply.

Cerebral embolism — A sudden blockage of a cerebral blood vessel by a clot travelling through and obstructing the vessel.

Cerebral haemorrhage — Bleeding into the brain tissue.

Cerebral infarction — Damage to an area of brain tissue caused by a sudden insufficiency of blood supply.

Cerebral thrombosis — Narrowing and eventual obstruction of a cerebral artery caused by accumulation of intravascular material of atheromatous origin.

Completed stroke — A stroke in which the clinical picture has become complete.

Cortical blindness — Loss of sight caused by lesions of the visual centre in the occipital lobe.

Dementia — Progressive mental and intellectual deterioration occurring over a period of time.

Diplopia — Seeing two images of a single object.

Dislocation — Disturbance of a normal relation of the bones forming a joint.

Drop attacks — Sudden falling to the ground, without warning and with no residual neurological signs. Usually caused by vertebro-basilar insufficiency.

Dysarthria — Defective speech caused by a disorder of articulation.

Dysphagia — Difficulty in swallowing.

Epilepsy — A paroxysmal transitory disturbance of brain function, ceasing spontaneously, with tendency to recur.

Hemianaesthesia — Loss of tactile sensation on one side of the body.

215

Hemianopia	Loss of vision in one half of the visual field in one or both eyes.	**Reflex**	An involuntary movement resulting from an afferent impulse, e.g. knee jerk.
Hemiplegia	Paralysis on one side of the body.	**RIND**	Reversible ischaemic neurological deficit (mini-stroke).
Hemiparesis	Muscular weakness (incomplete paralysis) on one side of the body.	**Spasticity**	A state of increased muscular tone with exaggerated tendon reflexes.
Homonymous hemianopia	Loss of vision in both right halves or both left halves of the visual field.	**Spatial sense**	Ability to appreciate position in space.
Lacunae	Small areas of softening in the brain tissue caused by tiny infarcts.	**Stroke**	An acute illness caused by a sudden cessation of blood supply to a part of the brain.
Monoparesis (monoplegia)	Muscular weakness or complete paralysis of one limb.	**Subarachnoid haemorrhage**	Bleeding into the subarachnoid space, usually caused by a burst vessel or aneurysm.
Papilloedema	Oedema of the optic disc caused by raised intracranial pressure or by diffuse retinal disease.	**Subclavian steal**	Reversal of the blood flow in the vertebral artery giving rise to symptoms of vertebrobasilar ischaemia.
Paraplegia	Paralysis of the lower limbs.		
Perseveration	Constant repetition of a meaningless word or phrase or repetition of a previously correct response, even after the response has become inappropriate.	**Subluxation (incomplete dislocation)**	Disarrangement of a joint in which the bony relationship is altered but contact between joint surfaces remains.
		TIA	Transient ischaemic attack.
Position sense	The ability to identify the position of a limb in space with eyes closed.	**Urinary incontinence**	Involuntary voiding of urine at an inappropriate time and in an inappropriate place.
Pseudobulbar palsy	Bilateral upper motor neurone (supranuclear) lesion of cranial nerves 9, 10 and 12.	**Vertigo**	A sensation of irregular swaying or spinning motion, either of oneself or of external objects and space.

REFERENCES

1. Gordon T, Sorlie P, Kannel WB. *The Framingham study: a 16-year follow-up.* Washington DC: US Government Printing Office, 1971.

2. MRC Working Party. MRC trial of drug treatment in mild hypertension. *Br Med J* 1985; **291:** 97–104.

3. Amery A, et al. Results of a trial by the European working party on hypertension in the elderly. *Lancet* 1978; **i:** 681–683.

4. Teasdale G, Jennett B. Assessment of coma and impaired consciousness, a practical scale. *Lancet* 1974; **ii:** 31–33.

5. Exton-Smith AN, Norton D, McLaren R. *An investigation of geriatric nursing problems in hospital.* National Corporation for the Care of Old People. London: Churchill Livingstone, 1975.

6. Henderson V. *The nature of nursing — a definition and its implications for practice, research and education.* New York: McMillan Company, 1966.

7. Goodglass H, Kaplan E. *The assessment of aphasia and related disorders.* London: Henry Kimpton, 1976.

8. Schuell H. *The Minnesota test for differential diagnosis of aphasia.* Minnesota: University of Minnesota Press, 1965.

9. Porch B. *The Porch index of communicative ability.* Palo Alto: Consulting Psychological Press, 1967.

10. Kertesz A, McCabe P. Recovery patterns and prognosis in aphasia. *Brain* 1977; **100:** 1–18.

11. Sarno MT, Silver MAM, Sands E. Speech therapy and language recovery in severe aphasia. *J Speech Hearing Dis* 1970; **13:** 607–623.

12. Hollond AL. *Communicative abilities in daily living: A test of function communication for aphasic adults.* University Park Press, 1980.

13. Mulley G. *Stroke — a handbook for the patient's family.* London: Chest, Heart and Stroke Association.

14. Isaacs B. *Understanding stroke illness.* London: Chest, Heart and Stroke Association.

15. Grasty P. *Home care for the stroke patient.* London: Chest, Heart and Stroke Association.

16. Veteran's Administration Co-operative Study Group in antihypertensive agents. Effects of treatment on morbidity in hypertension. *JAMA* 1967; **202:** 1028–1034, and *JAMA* 1970; **213:** 1143–1152.

SUGGESTED READING

Marshall J. *The management of cerebrovascular disease,* 3rd edn. Oxford: Blackwell Scientific Publications, 1976.

World Health Organisation. Stroke — treatment, rehabilitation and prevention. *WHO Chronicle* 1971; **25:** 466–469.

Working Group on Strokes. *Report of the Geriatric Committee of the Royal College of Physicians.* London: RCGP, 1974.

Weddell J, Beresford SA. *Planning for stroke patients. A four-year descriptive study of home and hospital care.* London: HMSO, 1979.

Todd JM. Physiotherapy in the early stages of hemiplegia. *Physiotherapy* 1974; **60** (11): 336–342.

Callum C. A patient after cerebrovascular accident. *Nurs Times* 1980; **76:** 1961–1964.

Draper J. Long-term care of the hemiplegic patient at home. *Nurs Mirror* 1974; **139:** 76–78.

Greenhalgh RM, Clifford Rose F, eds. *Progress in stroke research 2.* London: Pitman Publishing Limited, 1983.

Clifford Rose F, Capildeo R. *Stroke — the facts.* Oxford: Oxford University Press, 1983.

Lubbock G, ed. *Stroke care — an interdisciplinary approach.* London: Faber and Faber, 1983.

Hutchinson EC, Acheson EJ. *Strokes — natural history, pathology and surgical treatment.* Eastbourne: WB Saunders Company Ltd, 1975.

Marshall J, Briggs RSJ, Currie S. *Strokes*. London: Update Publications Ltd, 1982.

Bobath B. *Adult hemiplegia: evaluation and treatment*. 2nd edn. London: William Heinemann Medical Books Ltd, 1978.

Darnborough A, Kinrade D. *Directory for the disabled*. Cambridge: Woodhead Faulkner Ltd, 1981.

Hawker M. *Return to mobility: exercises for the stroke patient*. London: Chest, Heart and Stroke Association, 1978.

Law D, Paterson B. *Living after a stroke*. London: Souvenir Press, 1980.

Ritchie D. *Stroke — a diary of recovery*. London: Faber and Faber, 1974.

Gann R, Halves R. *Stroke*. 2nd edn. Southampton: Wessex Regional Library Information Service, 1983.

Disability rights handbook. London: Disability Alliance, published annually.

Dardier E. *The early stroke patient — positioning and movement*. Eastbourne: Baillière Tindall, 1980.

Mulley G. *Stroke — a handbook for the patient's family*. London: The Chest, Heart and Stroke Foundation, 1978.

Understanding strokes. London: South Camden Health Authority.

Self-help and the patient. A directory of national organisations concerned with various diseases and handicaps. London: The Patients Association, 8th edn, 1982.

Carr J, Shepherd R. *Early care of the stroke patient. A positive approach*. London: Heinemann Medical Books Ltd, 1979.

Jay P. *Help yourselves. Handbook for hemiplegics and their families*. Hornchurch, Essex: Ian Henry Publications, 1979.

Johnstone M. *The stroke patient. Principles of rehabilitation*. 1st edn. Edinburgh: Churchill Livingstone, 1978.

Publications by the Research Institute for Consumer Affairs (RICA): *Communication aids — a guide for people who have difficulty speaking; Aids for people with disabilities — a review of information services; Aids for people with disabilities — a bibliography with summaries of performance studies*. Available from: RICA, 14 Buckingham Street, London, WC2N 6DS.

Handling the handicapped. 1975. The Chartered Society of Physiotherapy, Woodhead–Faulkner Ltd, 7 Rose Crescent, Cambridge, CB2 3LL.

Gillingham FT, Mawdsley C, William AE, eds. *Stroke. Proceedings of the Ninth Pfizer International Symposium*. Edinburgh: Churchill Livingstone, 1976.

Mitchell JRA, Domenet JG, eds. *Thromboembolism — a new approach to therapy*. Report of a symposium organised by Geigy Pharmaceuticals. London: Academic Press, 1977.

Willoughby DA, Devon F, Cicala V, Malan E, eds. *Proceedings of the International Symposium on Arteriosclerosis*. Milan: Carlo Erba Foundation, 1973.

Eggers O. *Occupational therapy in the treatment of adult hemiplegia*. London: William Heinemann Medical Books Ltd, 1983.

Myco F. *Nursing care of the hemiplegic stroke patient*. London: Harper and Row, 1983.

Carr JH, Shepheard RB. *A motor relearning programme for stroke*. London: Heinemann Medical, 1982.

Mulley GP. *Practical management of stroke*. Beckenham: Croom Helm, 1984.

Editorial. Treatment of hypertension in the over-60s. *Lancet* 1985; **i**: 1369–1370.

Australian National Blood Pressure Study: treatment of mild hypertension in the elderly. *Med J Aust* 1981; **2**: 398–402.

Hypertension/Stroke Co-operative Study Group: effect of antihypertensive treatment on stroke recurrence. *JAMA* 1974; **229**: 409–418.

INDEX

Numbers in medium type indicate page numbers; those in **bold type** refer to figure and caption numbers.

Functional assessment 102
Fundus, hypertensive 93

G
Genetic factors, in stroke 8
Glenohumeral joint 237
Glioblastoma multiforme **131, 213**

H
Haematoma, subdural 62, 83, **128, 129, 199**
Haemorrhage
– cerebellar 42, 62
– cerebral 18
– intracerebral, unequal pupils in **82, 103**
– intracranial 17
– meningocerebral 67
– subarachnoid 41, 103, 216
– subhyaloid 94
Hand
– claw deformity 239
– hemiplegic 241
– muscle wasting in 99, 240
Head injury **127**
Heart
– block, complete **147**
– disease 7
Heel pads 302
Heel sores 297, 298, 300
Hemianaesthesia 215
Hemianopia 91, 215, **402**
Hemiparesis 110, 215
Hemiplegia 30, 84, 215
– arm, spasticity in **251**
– hand in **241**
– and sensory loss 147–148
Hemiplegic oedema **102, 103, 107**
Hemiplegic posture 259
Hoists 283
Home, patient at 201–211
– aids 202, **442–459**
– physiotherapy **462**
– problems 202
Horner's syndrome 89
Hydration 102
– maintaining 122
Hygiene
– maintaining personal 124
– oral 258, 288
Hypertension, treatment of 212–213
Hypertensive encephalopathy 62
Hypertensive fundus 93
Hypertrophy, ventricular **146**
Hypoxia 102
Hypothermia 62, **142**

I
Imaging, Doppler
– continuous wave 98
– pulsed 98
Incontinence sheath, condom urinary **314**
Infarct dementia, multiple 42, 61
Infarction
– boundary zone 42, **123**
– cerebral 17–18, **28**, 110, 173

– – acute 103
– myocardial **49**
Infections
– acute 62
– respiratory tract 109
– urinary tract 145
Intestinal obstruction **257**
Intracerebral haemorrhage, unequal pupils in **82, 103**
Intracranial haemorrhage 17
Intracranial thrombophlebitis 42
Investigations
– angiography 91–97
– – digital subtraction 98–100
– blood tests 70
– computerised axial tomography (CT scan) 86–90
– cranial echogram 85
– electrocardiogram 70–72
– echocardiography 73
– electroencephalography 74–81
– isotope brain scan 82–84, **175**
– non-invasive 98–100
– – carotid phonangiography 98
– – Doppler continuous wave imaging 98
– – Duplex scanning 98
– – oculoplethysmography 98
– – pulsed Doppler imaging 98
– – supraorbital Doppler recording 98
– in transient ischaemic attacks 103
Ischaemic attacks, transient (TIAs)
– cause of 41
– clinical features of 42
– management of 103–108
– – investigations 103
– treatment of 104, 213–214
– – drugs 104
– – surgery 104
– subclavian steal syndrome 42, **122**, 216
Ischaemic necrosis **256**
Isotope brain scan 82–84

K
Kitchen aids **397, 470**
Knee, x-ray of **252**

L
Lacunae 215
Lipids 70
Life processes, maintaining 122
– body temperature 122
– nursing observations 122
– nutrition and hydration 122
– respiration and cardiovascular function 122
Living, activities of daily 168–175
Lumen **19**
Lying **268, 269, 270**

M
Marsupial pads **313**
Meningioma **133, 214**
Meningocerebral haemorrhage 67
Metabolic disorders 62
Metastases
– multiple **134**
– pulmonary **136**

LIST OF USEFUL ORGANISATIONS

Action for Dysphasic Adults, Northcote House, 37A Royal Street, London SE1 7LL. Tel: 01–261 9572.

Age Concern, Bernard Sunley House, 60 Pitcairn Road, Mitcham, Surrey CR4 3LL. Tel: 01–640 5431.

Alzheimers Disease Society, Bank Buildings, Fulham Broadway, London SW6 1EP. Tel: 01–381 3177.

Association of Carers, first floor, 21/23 New Road, Chatham, Kent ME4 4QJ. Tel: 0634 813981.

Association of Continence Advisors, Disabled Living Foundation, 380/384 Harrow Road, London W9 2HU.

British Epilepsy Association, 3–6 Alfred Place, London WC1E 7EE. Tel: 01–580 2704.

British Geriatrics Society, 1 St Andrews Place, Regents Park, London NW1 4LB. Tel: 01–935 4004.

British Paraplegic Sports Society, Ludwig Guttman Sports Centre for the Disabled, Harvey Road, Aylesbury, Buckinghamshire. Tel: 0296 84848.

British Red Cross Society, 9 Grosvenor Crescent, London SW1X 7EJ. Tel: 01–235 5454.

Central Council for the Disabled, 25 Mortimer Street, London W1N 8AB. Tel: 01–637 5400.

Chest, Heart and Stroke Association, Tavistock House North, Tavistock Square, London WC1H 9JE. Tel: 01–387 3012.

College of Speech Therapists, 6 Lechmere Road, London NW2 5BU. Tel: 01–459 8521.

Community Service Volunteers, 237 Pentonville Road, London N1. Tel: 01–278 6601.

Disability Alliance, 25 Denmark Street, London WC2 8NJ. Tel: 01–240 0806.

Disabled Drivers' Association, Ashwellthorpe Hall, Ashwellthorpe, Norwich, Norfolk NOR 89W.

Disabled Living Foundation, 346 Kensington High Street, London W14 8NS. Tel: 01–289 6111.

Distressed Gentlefolks Aid Association, Vicarage Gate House, Vicarage Gate, London W8 4AQ. Tel: 01–229 9341.

EXTEND (Exercise Training for the Elderly and/or Disabled), 3 The Boulevard, Sheringham, Norfolk NR26 8LJ. Tel: 0263 822479.

Health Education Council, 78 New Oxford Street, London WC1A 1AH. Tel: 01–631 0930.

Hearing Aid Council, PO Box 153, 40A Ludgate Hill, London EC4M 7DE. Tel: 01–838 9226.

Help the Aged, 1 Sekforde Street, London EC1R 0BE. Tel: 01–253 0253.

Invalids at Home, Mrs S. Lomas, 17 Lepstone Gardens, Kenton, Middlesex. Tel: 01–907 1706.

Margaret Morris Movement, Suite 3/4, 39 Hope Street, Glasgow G2 6AG.

Methodist Homes for the Aged, Epworth House, 25/35 City Road, London EC1Y 1DR. Tel: 01–638 1431.

MIND (National Association for Mental Health), 22 Harley Street, London W1N 2ED. Tel: 01–637 0741.

Multiple Sclerosis Society, 25 Effie Road, London SW6. Tel: 01–736 6267.

National Institute of Adult Education, 35 Queen Anne Street, London W1. Tel: 01–580 3155.

Keep Fit Association, Upper Woburn Place, London WC1. Tel: 01–387 4349.

Patients' Association, 18 Charing Cross Road, London WC2 0HR. Tel: 01–240 0671.

Rehabilitation Engineering Movement Advisory Panels (REMAP), 25 Mortimer Street, London W1N 8AB. Tel: 01–637 5400.

Royal Association for Disability and Rehabilitation (RADAR), 25 Mortimer Street, London W1N 8AB. Tel: 01–637 5400.

Sexual Problems of the Disabled, 286 Camden Road, London N7 0BJ.

St John's Ambulance Brigade, 1 Grosvenor Crescent, London SW1X 7EF. Tel: 01–235 5231.

Society of Geriatric Nursing, 20 Cavendish Square, London W1M 0AB. Tel: 01–409 3333.

Talking Books Library, Mount Pleasant, Wembley, Middlesex HA0 1RR. Tel: 01–903 6666.

Taskforce, Pensioners Project, 287 Kingsland Road, London E8. Tel: 01–254 9674.

University of the Third Age, 6 Parkside Gardens, London SW19 5EJ. Tel: 01–636 8000.

Volunteer Stroke Scheme, Valerie Eaton Griffith (Organiser), St Martin's, Grimms Hill, Great Missenden, Bucks HP16 9BG.

WRVS (Women's Royal Voluntary Service), 17 Old Park Lane, London W1Y 4AJ. Tel: 01–499 6040.

Someone To Talk To Directory, compiled by Penny Webb, published by the Mental Health Foundation, 1985. Much useful information can be obtained from this comprehensive directory of self-help and community support agencies, national and local, in the UK and Republic of Ireland.

AIDS CENTRES

BELFAST Aids Centre, Rehabilitation Engineering Unit, Musgrave Park Hospital, Stockman's Lane, Belfast BT9 7JB. Tel: (0232) 669501.

BIRMINGHAM Disabled Living Centre, 260 Broad Street, Birmingham B1 2HF. Tel: 021-643 0980.

CAERPHILLY Aids and Information Centre, Wales Council for the Disabled, Caerbragdy, Industrial Estate, Bedwas Road, Caerphilly CF8 3SL. Tel: (0222) 887325.

EDINBURGH South Lothian Aids Distribution and Exhibition Centre, Astley Ainslie Hospital, Grange Loan, Edinburgh EH9 2HL. Tel: 031-447 9200, Exhibition Centre 031-447 6271.

LEEDS The William Merritt Disabled Living Centre, St Mary's Hospital, Greenhill Road, Armley, Leeds LS12 3QE. Tel: (0532) 793140.

LEICESTER: TRAIDS, 76 Clarendon Park Road, Leicester LE2 3AD. Tel: (0533) 700747.

LIVERPOOL Merseyside Aids Centre, Youens Way, East Prescott Road, Liverpool 14 2EP. Tel: 051-228 9221.

MANCHESTER Disabled Living Services, Redbank House, 4 St Chad's Street, Cheetham, Manchester M8 8QA. Tel: 061-832 3678.

NEWCASTLE UPON TYNE Newcastle upon Tyne Council for the Disabled, Aids Centre, Mea House, Ellison Place, Newcastle upon Tyne NE1 8XS. Tel: (0632) 323617.

SHEFFIELD Sheffield Aids Centre, Family and Community Services, 87/89 The Wicker, Sheffield S3 8HT. Tel: (0742) 737025.

SOUTHAMPTON Southampton Aids Centre, Southampton General Hospital, Tremona Road, Southampton SO9 4XY. Tel: (0703) 777222, ext. 3414 or 3233.

STOCKPORT Stockport Aids Centre, St Thomas Hospital, 59a Shaw Heath, Stockport SK3 8BL. Tel: 061-483 1010.

SWINDON Swindon Aids Centre, The Hawthorne Centre, Cricklade Road, Swindon, Wilts SN2 1AF. Tel: (0793) 37196.

WAKEFIELD National Demonstration Centre, Pinderfields Hospital, Aberford Road, Wakefield WF1 4DG. Tel: (0924) 375217, ext. 2510 or 2263.

SOME SUPPLIERS OF AIDS AND EQUIPMENT

Homecraft, 27 Trinity Road, London SW17 7SF. Tel: 01-672 7070.

Nottingham Medical Aids Ltd, Melton Road, West Bridgford, Nottingham NG2 6HD.

Anything Left-Handed Ltd, 65 Beak Street, London W1. Tel: 01-437 3910.

Dycem Ltd, Anti-Slip Division, Ashley Hill Trading Estate, Bristol BS2 9XS. Tel: 0272 559921.

Llewellyn and Co. Ltd, Carlton Works, Carlton Street, Liverpool L3 7ED. Tel: 051-236 5311.

SML Ltd, Bath Place, High Street, Barnet, Herts EN5 5XE. Tel: 01-440 6522.

Mullipel Fleeces, Bayer UK Ltd, Bayer House, Strawberry Hill, Newbury, Berkshire RG13 1JA. Tel: 0635 39000. (Range of fleeces for prevention of pressure sores.)

Medical-Assist Ltd, Commerce Way, Whitehall Industrial Estate, Colchester, Essex CO2 8HH. Tel: 0206 45242. (Urinary drainage systems.)

Robinsons of Chesterfield, Wheat Bridge, Chesterfield, Derbyshire S40 2AD. Tel: 0246 31101. (Incontinence pads and pants.)

Astec Environmental Systems Ltd, 31 Lynx Crescent, Weston Industrial Estate, Weston-super-Mare, Avon BS24 9DJ. Tel: 0934 418685. (Clinifloat mattresses for prevention and treatment of pressure sores and for care of incontinent patients.)

Vernon-Carus Ltd, Penwortham Mills, Preston, Lancashire PR1 9SN. Tel: 0772 744493/8. (Incontinence pads and pants.)

Coloplast Ltd, Orchard Lane, Huntingdon, Cambridgeshire PE18 6QT. Tel: 0480 55451. (Aids for management of urinary incontinence.)